MIASMA

The Road Less Travelled

Dr Harsh Nigam
MBBS, MD, MF (HOM)

B. JAIN PUBLISHERS (P) LTD.
USA — EUROPE — INDIA

MIASMA

First Edition: 2012
2nd Impression: 2017

All rights reserved. No part of this book may be reproduced, stored in a retrieval system or transmitted, in any form or by any means, mechanical, photocopying, recording or otherwise, without any prior written permission of the publisher.

© with the publisher

Published by Kuldeep Jain for
B. JAIN PUBLISHERS (P) LTD.
D-157, Sector-63, NOIDA-201307, U.P. (INDIA)
Tel.: +91-120-4933333 • *Email:* info@bjain.com
Website: **www.bjain.com**
Registered office: 1921/10, Chuna Mandi, Paharganj,
New Delhi-110 055 (India)

Printed in India by
J.J. Offset Printers

ISBN: 978-81-319-1921-7

DEDICATION

This work is dedicated first and foremost to my guru Paramhans Baba Ram Mangal Das of Ayodhya, also to all the masters of Homoeopathy specially Hahnemann, Kent, Allen, Roberts, Foubister, Patterson, Ortega, Paschero, Vannier, Banerjea, for me they are the 'illuminati' of Homoeopathy.

Through the ages since inception of Homoeopathy they have lit the true path to the treatment of chronic diseases, by their wisdom.

I bow to them.

THE FOUNDATION OF ALL TRUE WISDOM:

γωυθι σεαυτδν*

*KNOW YOURSELF

Footnote, Para 141, Hahnemann. S., The Organon Of Medicine

'If I have seen a little further it is by standing on the shoulders of Giants.' *

—Issac Newton

* Scientific progress is a cumulative process, in which each generation of scientists builds on the discoveries of its predecessors: a collaborative march - gradual, methodical, unstopable - towards a greater understanding of the natural laws that govern the universe.

FOREWORD

A good Homeopathic physician is an asclepiad who knows he is an instrument, that his duty is to keep his patient free from miasmatic affections which hinder the enjoyment of individuality and that his sacred mission is to preserve health.

The miasm represent everything that has been super imposed on the essential being of an individual whether from environment or acquired by error, they also represent a false personality that is a personality which does not correspond faithfully to his intimate essential nature.

Deformation of the natural symptoms or symptom patterns are causes by suppressive therapeutics and sometime due to enantiopathic, allopathic or pseudo homeopathic therapies which stimulate miasmatic episodes, hence it is essential to know the miasmas.

The homeopathic remedy, that is the true simillimum prescribed one after another through time will liberate this essential nature of man and reintegrate it back to harmony thus it stimulates and impels the individual towards true cure.

Dr. Harsh Nigam's object is to expose why knowledge of miasm is essential and how to know the basic background of all chronic diseases and thereby give the incurable disease a perfect "TRUE CURE". I hope that all the student of homeopathy will get the pleasure of true cure of chronic diseases, by the help of this work which is timely, crisp and clear in content keeping the true dynamic thought of concept of miasma alive and co-relating it beautifully with modern concepts specially immunity.

Dr. Jagdish Chandra Nigam
B.M.S. (Lucknow),
D.F. Hom. (London),
P.G.G.F.H. (Glasgow),
P.G.G.F.H. (Germany).

ACKNOWLEDGEMENT

I offer my humble gratitude to my parents Mrs. Shobha & Dr. Jagdish Chandra Nigam. I owe everything in my life and in Homoeopathy to them.

None of my days would have been complete without my wife Dr. Prachi and son Virat, to them my thanks for being there.

A special thanks to Shri Sanjay Jain for managing the clinic so well that I have time to write book and do some free thinking.

In writing this work I have heavily borrowed from excellent works of Hahnemann, Kent, Allen, Roberts, Pashero, Ortega, Swan, Vannier, Banerjea etc.

In the task of delivering Materia Medica of nosodes with out missing the crux of matter I am indebted to my student Dr. Monika Singh and Dr. Dinanath Yadav.

For the patient and thorough editorial assistance I thank Mr. Rakesh Kapoor. I also thank Dr. Devesh Sachan for acting as spell check. To Dr. Priyanka Shukla, I must say that her suggestion and criticism of what has remained unfinished, spurred a last minute burst of pen, adding new insight into the Materia Medica of *Carcinosin*, I thank you all. I also thank Dr. Preeti for her help.

PREFACE

As sentient beings, it is human nature to seek meaning. Each successive generation takes up this search within the accumulated knowledge of their era and the limits of their experience. This quest for meaning has returned again and again to the issues of life, death and the nature of illness.

In this century the developing world has often looked to the sciences [most notably genetics and quantum theory] for answers to metaphysical questions.

Although the weight of experimental evidence has vindicated this reductionist approach for many material problems, the negative consequence of this approach has been the tendency to reject models, which appear, at first glance, to be non-scientific. An eminent geneticist, for example, recently pronounced that infants with limb agenesis born to thalidomide mothers could not have an inherited basis, since there was no explanation in genetic theory for this. The arrogance of medical science is that it often subverts those empirical observations that it cannot accommodate.

In the latter half of the 20th century this rejection has extended to many homoeopathic tenets, [for e.g. activity of ultra molecular potencies and miasm theory, for example] The criticism of orthodox science is often justified, because many opportunities for information-gathering and sound scientific enquiry have been squandered by the homoeopathic medical community itself. On the other hand, the thought that scientific proof is definitive in medicine can exclude many valuable, but empirical treatments in an era when science is not yet equipped to test the hypothesis of dynamic aspect of homoeopathy.

In this book we will examine one of Homoeopathy's holy grail, - miasm theory. Before we relegate the theory of miasms to the history books, we will re-examine the trains of thought, which over the last two centuries, have sought to explain the nature of chronic illness. After we have looked at miasm theory in its historical context we must then ask if there are human or animal phenomena to which these models might still usefully be applied.

A theory that supports non-genetic transmission might yet arise from accumulated clinical experience. The concept of a non-genetic trait, transferred from one generation to the next, is particularly interesting and controversial.

During subsequent proof reading of this work by my select students, it came to my notice that this work has become very dense I have always believed that the concept of miasma opens to your mind as you grow in your practice of the rationale treatment of chronic diseases by homoeopathy.

So what happens to the beginner in Homoeopathy? To them I shall suggest a plan of study of this book.

Read section, I and section II thoroughly. Section III would Simulate modern medical student and would give some modern explanation to the concept of miasma.

There after the book shall cater differently to different set of readers.

First for the student who is under graduate: After reading section I,II,III, thereafter read section V followed by section VII.

Secondly for the postgraduate student: grasp whole of section IV and section V then study section VII. In your OPD's apply section VI on cases and analyse the results.

Lastly to the reader who is adapt in homoeopathy: I shall implore to study and ponder upon section IV the potential Study of miasma section VI miasmatic case management because it shall give them ideas and tips from past masters on how to tackle Chronic disease. To the adept I would also urge to study the entire Materia Medica of five nosode especially *Carcinosin*. This Materia Medica of nosodes would be of high degree of practical use in their clinical work.

PUBLISHER'S NOTE

Dr Harsh Nigam is one of great authors we have with us at B. Jain. His knowledge of clinical subjects and homeopathy is commendable and the balance he maintains in these aspects makes him one of the most wonderful prescribers in today's time. He has carried the heritage of homeopathy from his father Dr Jagdish Chandra Nigam who is also a homeopathic master practitioner and well known in the field of homeopathy. Dr Jagdish learnt with the pioneers of our field like Foubister, Blackie, Twentymann, Leddermann and Margaret Tyler, and passed on all his learning's to his son Dr Harsh Nigam. What we get in Dr Harsh's books is the knowledge passed from the pioneers to Dr Jagdish and then to Dr Harsh and at that level it is enriched with his analytical mind and experience and is made available to the readers. His book on Case Taking is a beautiful example of culmination of different ways of case taking. Dr Harsh has considered and given a practical insight into what is best of different ways of Case Taking and how to apply same. Now comes his comprehensive work on miasms, which is one of the most misunderstood and misinterpreted topic in homeopathy. Dr Harsh has meticulously analyzed majority of the work done on miasma and has explained how to find the correct miasma of a patient and treat it so as to make a true cure possible. His straightforward way of explaining the aspects given by various teachers like Hahnemann, Kent, Ortega, Roberts, and alike makes the task of understanding the concept of miasma, possible. We hope that all students of homeopathy pay attention to this work and absorb it and apply it for bringing better and finer results with this gentle science of healing.

Kuldeep Jain
C.E.O., B. Jain Publishers (P) Ltd.

CONTENTS

Dedication	iii
Foreword	v
Acknowledgement	vi
Preface	vii
Publisher's Note	xii

SECTION I: HISTORICAL PERSPECTIVE

1. A Reminder from Hahnemann (Written 200 Years Ago) — 2
2. Hahnemann's Logical Deduction of Miasma — 7
3. Why Hahnemann Thought of Miasma — 22
4. Why Should We Know Miasma — 28

SECTION II: THEORY OF MIASMA AFTER HANNEMANN

5. Hahnemann, Samuel — 35
6. Allen, J.H. — 39
7. Kent, James Tyler — 42
8. Roberts, H.A. — 44
9. Paschero, T.P.[2] — 46
10. Eizayaga and Ortega — 47
11. Julian, O.A. — 48
12. H. Montfort-Cabello — 49
13. Sankaran, Rajan — 50
14. Nigam, Harsh — 51
15. Current Understanding of Miasma — 53

SECTION III: IMMUNITY & MIASMA

16. Concepts of Immune System — 56
17. Concept of Immunologic Balance — 69
18. Immunity & Diseases — 73
19. Immunity and Homoeopathy — 80

SECTION IV: POTENTIAL STUDY OF MIASMA

20. Before Understanding Potential Aspect of Miasm — 104
21. Proposed Psoric Theory of Disease — 106
22. Bond of Psora with Life Forces — 109
23. The Potential Study of Miasmatics — 112
24. Degree of Activity of Miasm — 115
25. The Miasmatic Potential — 116
26. Inhibitory Points — 119
27. The Nature of Miasm Latent & Chronic — 126

SECTION V: MIASMA AS DISEASE CAUSATIVE FORCE

28. Inquiry into the Process of Disease Phenomenon — 134
29. Hahnemann's Causative Classification of Disease — 139
30. Suppression of Miasma — 140
31. The Eizayaga Model of Layers of Disease — 160
32. How to Recognize Miasma by Symptomatology — 165
33. Key Characteristics of Miasma — 189

SECTION VI: MIASMATIC CASE MANAGEMENT

34. Hahnemannian Model of Anti-Miasmatic Treatment — 200
35. P.N. Banerjee on Miasmatic Case Management — 203
36. Miasmatic Prescribing — 207

SECTION VII: MATERIA MEDICA STUDIES

37. Overview — 213
38. Psorinum — 216
39. Medorrhinum — 237
40. Syphilinum — 255
41. Tuberculinum — 274
42. Carcinosin — 283

BIBLIOGRAPHY — 304

SECTION I: HISTORICAL PERSPECTIVE

Chapter: 1
A Reminder from Hahnemann

Chapter: 2
Hahnemann's Logical Deduction of Miasma

Chapter: 3
Why Hahnemann Thought of Miasma

Chapter: 4
Why Should we Know Miasma

Chapter 1

A Reminder from Hahnemann[15] (Written 200 Years Ago)

As long as accurate observation, unprejudiced research, and careful comparison have failed to demonstrate really constant primary maladies for the amazing number of morbid phenomena and cases of disease occurring in the human subject, which nature appears to produce in endless variety and very dissimilar to one another, so long evidently must every single disease as it occurs be homoeopathically treated according to the array of symptoms that show themselves in each case.

According to the medical teachers and their books: "What do we care about the presence of many other diverse symptoms that are observable in the case of disease. The physician should pay no attention to such empirical trifles; his practical tact, the penetrating glance of his mental eye into the hidden nature of the malady, enables him to determine at the very first sight of the patient what is the matter with him, what pathological form of disease he has to do with, and what name he has to give it, and his therapeutic knowledge teaches him what prescription he must order for it."

Thus then were prepared by pathology those illusory pictures of disease which were transferred lege artis to the patient, and falsely attributed to him, and thus it was rendered it so easy for the physician to recall to his memory without hesitation a couple of prescriptions which the clinical therapeutics [of the prescription manual] had in readiness, for this name.

Shall the pernicious jugglery of routine treatment still continue to exist? Shall the symptoms of the patient, that is the account of his sufferings, vainly resound through the air unheard by his doctor, without exciting any helpful attention of any human heart?

Or can the so remarkably different complaints and sufferings of each single patient indicate anything else than the peculiarity of his disease? If not, what can this distinct voice of nature, which expresses itself in terms so appropriate to the various symptoms of the patient, what can it mean if not to render his morbid state as cognizable as possible to the sympathizing and attentive physician, in order to enable him to distinguish the very minutest shades of difference of this case from every other?

The patient reveals to the observer, by words and signs, the great variety of his altered sensations and morbid actions. The disease, being but a peculiar condition, cannot speak, cannot tell its own story; the patient suffering from it can alone render an account of his disease by the various signs of his disordered health, the sufferings he feels, the symptoms he can complain of, and by the alterations in him that are perceptible to the senses.

The pseudo-wisdom of the ordinary physicians thinks all these symptoms are scarcely worth listening to; and even if they listen to it, they allege that it is of no importance, that it is empirical and expressed in a very unlearned manner by nature, that it does not coincide with what their pathological books teach them, and is, therefore, not for their purpose, but in place thereof they put forward a figment of their learned reveries as the picture of the internal [never ascertainable] state of the disease, in their folly they substitute this delusive pathological picture for the individual state of each case of disease.

Since the internal operations and processes of the living human organism cannot be inspected, either in the healthy or yet in the diseased state, and on that very account all deductions from the exterior respecting the interior are deceptive, and as the knowledge of disease can be neither a metaphysical problem nor the product of fantastic speculation, but is an affair of pure experience by the senses, because disease as a manifestation, can only be apprehended by observations. Careful observation finds every individual case of disease in nature to differ from every other. (With the exception of such diseases that are caused by a miasm of constant character). No name borrowed from a pathological system should be attached to morbid states, which in reality differ so much among themselves.

Diseases are nothing more than alterations of the sound, normal state of health so there can be for the physician no other true view of diseases which shall enable him to discover what should be the aim of his treatment and what there is to be cured, except what is perceived by the senses of the observable alterations of health in the patient.

The honest physician, whose earnest desire it is to investigate the peculiar character of the disease before him, I say, will observe his patient minutely, with all his senses, will make the patient and his attendants detail all his sufferings and symptoms, and will carefully note, them down without adding anything to or taking anything from them; he will thus have a faithful genuine picture of the disease, and along with that an accurate knowledge of all there is in it to be cured and removed; he will then have a true knowledge of the disease.

Now, as disease can be nothing more than alterations of the sound, normal state of health, and as every alteration of the health of a healthy person is disease, so cure can be nothing but transformation of the abnormal state of health into the normal and healthy state.

If, medicines are the agents for curing diseases, they must, possess the power of effecting an alteration in the state of health.

The most zealous efforts of one who devotes himself to the cure of diseases [a physician], must hence, before all things, be directed to obtain a foreknowledge of those properties and actions of medicines by means of which he may effect the cure or amelioration of every individual case of disease with the greatest certainty.

Now, it is impossible that the alterations in man's health which medicines are capable of producing, can be ascertained and observed more purely, certainly, and completely, by any other method in the world, than by the action of medicines upon healthy individuals; indeed, there is no other way besides this conceivable, in which it were possible to obtain experience that shall be at all of an accurate character respecting the real alterations they are capable of effecting in man's health.

For the action they show with chemical reagents reveals only chemical properties, which are no clue to their power over the living human organism. The alterations they produce when given to animals only teach what they can do them each according to its nature, would effect on man, endowed as he is with an organization of a perfectly different character, and with very different powers both of mind and body. Even when given in human diseases in order to ascertain their effects, the peculiar symptoms which were solely due to the medicine can never be distinctly recognized, never accurately distinguished, amid the turmoil of the morbid symptoms already present, so as to admit of our ascertaining which of the changes effected were owing to the medicine, which to the disease.

The simple natural way alone remains for us, in order to ascertain clearly, purely, and with certainty, the powers of medicines upon man, that is, the alterations they are capable of effecting on his health-the only, genuine and simple natural way, viz. to administer the medicines to healthy individuals.

The physician must possess the most perfect knowledge possible of the pure alterations in the health produced on the healthy human body by the greatest possible number of single medicines, before he ventures to undertake, the administration of medicines to a sick person for his disease.

Chapter 2

Hahnemann's Logical Deduction of Miasma[15]

The Homoeopathic healing art, as taught in my own writings and in those of my pupils, when faithfully followed, has shown its natural superiority over any allopathic treatment in a very decided and striking manner; and this not only in those diseases which, suddenly attack men [the acute diseases], but also in epidemic diseases and in sporadic fevers.

Venereal diseases also have been radically healed by Homoeopathy much more surely, without disturbing or destroying the local manifestation healing the internal fundamental disease from within only, through the best specific remedy.

Even in these other kinds of non-venereal chronic diseases, by following the teachings presented in my former writings and my former, oral lectures, accomplished far more than all the other methods of curing; i.e., when they found the patient not too much run down and spoiled by allopathic treatment.

Using the more natural treatment, Homoeopathic physicians have frequently been able in a short time to remove the chronic disease which they had before them, after examining it according to all the symptoms perceptible to the senses; and the means of cure were the most suitable among the Homoeopathic remedies, used in their small doses which had been so far proved as to their pure, true effects.

The complaints yielded mostly to very small doses of that remedy which had proved its ability to produce the same series of morbid symptoms in the healthy body; and, if the disease was not altogether too inveterate and had not been too much and in too great a degree mismanaged by allopathy, it often yielded for a considerable time.

But some gross errors of diet, taking cold, the change of weather and then some violent exertion of the body or mind, repeated fright, great grief, sorrow and continuous vexation, often caused in a weakened body the re-appearance of one or more of the ailments which seemed to have been already overcome.

This new condition was often aggravated by some quite new concomitants, which if not more threatening than the former ones which had been removed homoeopathically were often just as troublesome and now more obstinate.

This would be especially the case whenever the seemingly cured disease had for its foundation a psora, which had been more fully developed. When such a relapse would take place the Homoeopathic physician would give the remedy most fitting among the medicines then known, as if directed against a new disease, and this would again be attended by a pretty good success, which for the time would again bring the patient into a better state.

As in the former case, however, in which merely the troubles which seemed to have been removed were renewed, the remedy which had been serviceable the first time would prove less useful, and when repeated again it would help still less.

Homoeopathic remedies served at last hardly even as weak palliatives. But usually, after repeated attempts to conquer the disease which appeared in a form always somewhat changed.

Thus there ever followed varying complaints ever more troublesome, and, as time proceeded, more threatening, and this even while the mode of living was correct and with a punctual observance of directions. The chronic disease could, despite all efforts, be but little delayed in its progress by the Homoeopathic physician and grew worse from year to year.

This was, and remained, the quicker or slower process in such treatments in all non-venereal, severe chronic diseases, even when these were treated in exact accordance with the Homoeopathic art. Their beginning was promising, the continuation less favorable, the outcome hopeless.

Why was this unfavorable result of the continued treatment of the non-venereal chronic diseases even by Homoeopathy?

What was the reason of the thousands of unsuccessful endeavors to heal the other diseases of chronic nature so that lasting health might result?

Might this be caused, by too small number of Homoeopathic remedial means that have so far been proved as to their pure action?

The followers of Homoeopathy have thus consoled themselves. This excuse, never satisfied the founder of Homoeopathy, particularly because even the new additions of proved valuable medicines, have not advanced the healing of chronic [non-venereal] diseases by single-step.

While acute diseases [unless these, at their commencement, threaten unavoidable death] are not only passably removed, by means of correct application of Homoeopathic remedies, but with the assistance of the never-resting, preservative vital force in our organism, find a speedy and complete cure.

Why, this vital force cannot, efficiently affect any true and lasting recovery in these chronic maladies even with the aid of the Homoeopathic remedies which best cover their present symptoms, while this same force which is created for the restoration of our organism is nevertheless so successfully active in completing the recovery even in severe acute diseases? What is there to prevent this?

The answer to this question, which is so natural, inevitably led me to the discovery of the nature of these chronic diseases.

To find out then the reason why all the medicines known to Homoeopathy failed to bring a real cure in the chronic non-venereal diseases, and to gain an insight into the true nature of the thousands of chronic diseases which still remain uncured, despite the truth of the Homoeopathic Law of Cure, this very serious task has occupied me since the years 1816 and 1817, night and day.

It was a continually repeated fact that the non-venereal chronic diseases, after being time and again removed homoeopathically by the remedies fully proved up to the present time, always returned in a more or less varied form and with new symptoms, or reappeared annually with an increase of complaints.

This fact gave me the first clue that the Homoeopathic physician with such a chronic [non-venereal] case, has not only to combat the disease presented before his eyes and he must not view and treat it as if it were a well-defined disease, but that he has always to encounter only some separate fragment of a more deep-seated original disease.

The great extent of this disease is shown in the new symptoms appearing from time to time; so that the Homoeopathic physician must not hope to permanently heal the separate manifestations of this kind in the presumption, that they are well- defined, separately existing diseases which can be healed permanently and completely.

He, therefore, must first find out as far as possible the whole extent of all the accidents and symptoms belonging to the unknown primitive malady, before he can hope to discover one or more medicines which may homoeopathically cover the whole of the original disease by means of its peculiar symptoms.

By this method he may then be able to victoriously heal and wipe out the malady in its whole extent, that is, all the fragments of a disease appearing in so many various forms.

The original malady sought for, must be of a miasmatic chronic nature. This clearly appeared to me from the fact, that after the disease has once advanced and developed to a certain degree it can never be removed by the strength of robust constitution, it can never be overcome by the most wholesome diet and order of life, nor will it die out of itself.

It is even more aggravated, from year to year, through a transition into other and more serious symptoms, even till the end of his life, like every other chronic, miasmatic sickness; e.g., the venereal bubo which has not been healed from within by mercury, its specific remedy, this chronic non-venereal disease, also, never passes away of itself, but, even with the most correct mode of life and with the most robust bodily constitution and it increases every year and unfolds even more into new and worse symptoms, to the end of man's life.

I had come thus far in my investigations and observations with such non-venereal patients, the obstacle to the cure of many cases which seemed like well defined disease seemed very often to lie in a former eruption of itch, which was frequently not confessed; and the beginning of all the subsequent sufferings usually dated from that time.

After a careful inquiry it usually turned but that little traces of it [small pustules of itch, herpes, etc.] had showed themselves with them from time to time, even if but rarely, as an undoubtful sign of a former infection of this kind.

These circumstances, in connection with the fact that innumerable observations of physicians, and my own experience, had shown that an eruption of itch suppressed by faulty practice or one which had disappeared from the skin through other means was evidently followed, in persons otherwise healthy, by the same or similar symptoms; these circumstances, I repeat, could leave no doubt in my mind as to the internal foe which I had to combat in my medical treatment of such cases.

Gradually I discovered more effective means against this original malady that caused so many complaints; against this malady which may be called by the general name of Psora; i.e., the internal itch disease with or without its attendant eruption on the skin.

Most painstaking observations as to the aid afforded by the antipsoric remedies which were added in the first of these eleven years have taught me evermore, how frequently not only the moderate, but also the more severe and the most severe, chronic diseases are of this origin.

I was thus instructed by my continued observations, comparisons and experiments in the last years, that the ailments and infirmities of body and soul, which, in their manifest complaints, differ so radically and which, with different patients, appear so very unlike [if they do not belong to the two venereal diseases, syphilis and sycosis], are but partial manifestations of the ancient miasma of leprosy and itch; i.e., merely descendants of one and the same vast original malady, Psora.

In Europe and also on the other continents so far as it is known, according to all investigations, only three chronic miasms are found, the diseases caused by which manifest themselves through local symptoms, and from which most, of not all, the chronic diseases originate; namely, first, SYPHILIS, which I have also called the venereal chancre disease; then SYCOSIS, or the fig-wart disease, and finally the chronic disease which lies at the foundation of the eruption of itch; i.e., the PSORA: which I shall treat of first as the most important.

PSORA is that most ancient, most universal, most destructive, and yet most misapprehended chronic miasmatic disease which for many thousands of years has disfigured and tortured mankind, and which during the last centuries has become the mother of all the thousands of incredibly various Acute and Chronic [non-venereal] diseases, by which the whole civilized human race on the inhabited globe is being more and more afflicted.

PSORA is the oldest miasmatic chronic disease known to us. Just as tedious as syphilis and sycosis, and therefore not to be extinguished before the last breath of the longest human life, unless it is thoroughly cured, since not even the most robust constitution is able to destroy and extinguish it by its own proper strength, Psora, or the Itch disease, is beside this the oldest and most hydra-headed of all the chronic miasmatic diseases.

So great a flood of numberless nervous troubles, painful ailments, spasms, ulcers [cancers], adventitious formations, dyscrasias, paralysis, consumptions and crippling of soul, mind and body were never seen in ancient times when the Psora mostly confined itself to its dreadful cutaneous symptom leprosy. Only during the last few centuries has mankind been flooded with these infirmities, owing to the causes just mentioned.

It was thus that PSORA became the most universal mother of chronic diseases.

The psora, which is now so easily and so rashly robbed of its ameliorating cutaneous symptom, the eruption of itch, which acts vicariously for the internal disease, has been producing within the last three hundred years more and more secondary symptoms and indeed so many that at least seven-eighths of all the chronic maladies spring from it as their only source, while the remaining eighth springs from syphilis and sycosis or from a complication of two of these three miasmatic chronic diseases or from a complication of all three of them.

Even syphilis, which on account of its easy curability yields to the smallest dose of the best preparation of mercury, and sycosis, which on account of the slight difficulty in its cure through a few doses of *Thuja* and *Nitric acid* in alternation, only pass into a tedious malady difficult to cure when they are complicated with psora.

Thus PSORA is among all diseases the one, which is most misapprehended, and, therefore, has been medically treated in the worst and most injurious manner.

The diseases, partly acute but chiefly chronic, springing from such a one-sided destruction of the chief skin-symptom [eruption and itching] which acts vicariously and assuages the internal Psora.

Psora then shows itself from within in a thousand different diseases. The disease then sooner or later return with the malady following such a treatment; e.g. with swellings obstinate pains in one part or another, with hypochondriac or hysterical troubles, gout, consumption, tubercular phthisis, continual or spasmodic asthma, blindness, deafness, paralysis, caries of the bones, ulcers (cancer), spasms, hemorrhages, diseases of the mind and soul, etc.,

The physicians imagine that they have before them something entirely new and treat it again and again and according to the old routine of their therapeutics in a useless and harmful manner, directing their medicines against phantom disease; i.e. against causes invented by them for the ailments as they appear, until the patient, after many years' suffering continually aggravated, is at last freed from their hands by death, the end of all earthly maladies.

[Hahnemann elucidates many examples and then states further]

Who, after meditating on even these few examples would remain so thoughtless as to ignore the great evil hidden within, the Psora, of which evil the eruption of itch and its other forms, the Tinea capitis, milk crust, tetter, etc., are only indications announcing the internal, monstrous disease of the whole organism, only local external symptoms which act vicariously and mitigating for the internal disease? Who, after reading even the few cases described, would hesitate to acknowledge that the Psora, as already stated, is the most destructive of all chronic miasmas? All such miasmas become first internal maladies of the whole system before their external assuaging symptom appears on the skin.

We shall more closely elucidate this process, and in consequence we shall see that all miasmatic maladies which show peculiar local ailments on the skin are always present as internal maladies in the system before they show their local symptom externally upon the skin; but that only in acute diseases, after taking their course through a certain number of days, the local symptom, together with the internal disease, is to disappear, which then leaves the body free from both.

In chronic miasmas, however, the outer local symptom may either be driven from the skin or may disappear of itself, while the internal disease, if uncured, neither in whole nor in part ever leaves the system; on the contrary, it continually increases with the years, unless healed by proper internal medicines.

With respect to the origin of these three chronic maladies, as in the acute miasmatic eruptional diseases, three different important moments are to be more attentively considered:

1. The time of infection;
2. The period of time during which the whole organism is being penetrated by the disease infused, until it has developed within;
3. The breaking out of the external ailment, whereby nature externally demonstrates the completion of the internal development of the Miasmatic malady throughout the whole organism.

The infection with miasmas, as well of the acute as of the above mentioned chronic diseases, takes place, without doubt, in one single moment, and that moment is the one most favorable for infection.

Does it not take ten to twelve days after infection with smallpox, before the inflammatory fever and the outbreak of the smallpox on the skin take place?

What has nature been doing with the infection received in these ten or twelve days? Was it not necessary to first embody the disease in the whole organism before nature was enabled to kindle the fever, and to bring out the eruption on the skin?

Measles also require ten or twelve days after infection or inoculation before this eruption with its fever appears. After infection with scarlet fever seven days usually pass before the scarlet fever, with the redness of the skin, breaks out.

What then did nature do with the received miasma during the intervening days? What else but to incorporate the whole disease of measles or scarlet fever in the entire living organism before she had completed the work, so as to be enabled to produce the measles and the scarlet fever with their eruption.

From the progress of all these miasmatic diseases we may plainly see that, after the contagion from exterior, the malady connected with it in the interiors of the whole man must first be developed; i.e., the whole interior man must first have become thoroughly sick of smallpox, measles or scarlet fever, before these various eruptions can appear on the skin.

For all these acute miasmatic diseases the human constitution possesses that process which, as a rule, is so beneficent to wipe them out in the course of two to three weeks, through a kind of crisis, from the organism so that man then is to be entirely healed in a short time, unless he be killed by them.

In the chronic miasmatic diseases nature observes the same course with respect to the mode of contagion and the antecedent formation of the internal disease, before the external declarative symptoms of its internal completion manifests itself on the surface of the body. The great remarkable difference from the acute diseases is that in the chronic miasmata the entire internal disease, as we have mentioned before, remains in the organism during the whole life, and it increases with every year, if it is not exterminated and thoroughly cured by homoeopathic art.

Of these chronic miasmata I shall for this purpose only adduce those two, which we know somewhat more exactly; namely, the venereal chancre and the itch.

In impure coition there arises, most probably at the very moment in the spot that is touched and rubbed, the specific contagion.

If this contagion has taken effect, then the whole living body is ill with it. Immediately after the moment of contagion the formation of the venereal disease in the whole of the interior begins.

In that part of the sexual organs where the infection has taken place, nothing unnatural is noticed in the first days, nothing diseased, inflamed or corroded; so also all washing and cleansing of the parts immediately after the impure coition is in vain. The spot remains healthy according to appearance, only the internal organism is called into activity by the infection so as to incorporate the venereal miasma and to become thoroughly diseased with the venereal malady.

Only when this penetration of all the organs by the disease caught has been effected, only when the whole being has been changed into a man entirely venereal, i.e., when the development of the venereal disease has been completed, only then diseased nature endeavors to mitigate the internal evil and to soothe it, by producing a local symptom which first shows itself as a vesicle [usually in the spot originally infected], and later breaks out into a painful ulcer called the chancre; this does not appear before five, seven or fourteen days, sometimes, though rarely, not before three, four or five weeks after the infection. This is therefore manifestly a chancre ulcer which acts vicariously for the internal malady, and which has been produced from within by the organism after it has become venereal through and through, and is able through its touch to communicate also to other men the same miasma; i.e., the venereal disease.

Now, if the entire disease thus arising is again extinguished through the internally given specific remedy, then the chancre also is healed and the man recovers.

But if the chancre is destroyed through local applications before the internal disease is healed, the miasmatic chronic venereal disease remains in the organism as syphilis, and it is aggravated, if not then cured internally, from, year to year until the end of man's life, even the most robust constitution being unable to annihilate it within itself.

Only through the cure of the venereal disease, which pervades the whole internal of the body [as I have taught and practiced for many years], the chancre and its local symptom, will also simultaneously be cured in the most effective manner; and this is best effected without the use of any external application for its removal.

Psora [itch disease] is chronic non-venereal disease and like syphilis its original development is similar.

The itch disease is, however, also the most contagious of all chronic miasmata, far more infectious than the other two chronic miasmata, the venereal chancre disease and the fig-wart disease. The disposition of being affected with the miasma of itch is found with almost everyone and under almost all circumstances, which is not the case with the other two miasmata.

As soon as the miasma of itch, e.g., touches the hand, in the moment when it has taken effect, it no more remains local. Henceforth all washing and cleansing of the spot avail nothing. Nothing is seen on the skin during the first days; it remains unchanged, and, according to appearance, healthy. There is no eruption or itching to be noticed on the body during these days, not even on the spot infected.

The nerve which was first affected by the miasma has already communicated it in all invisible dynamic manner to the nerves of the rest of the body, and the living organism has been compelled to appropriate this miasma gradually to itself until the change of the whole being to be thoroughly psoric, and thus the internal development of the Psora, has reached completion.

Only when the whole organism feels itself transformed by this peculiar chronic-miasmatic disease, the diseased vital force endeavors to alleviate and to soothe the internal malady through the establishment of a suitable local symptom on the skill, the itch-vesicles. So long as this eruption continues, in its normal form, the internal psora, with its secondary ailments, cannot break forth, but must remain covered, slumbering, latent and bound.

Usually it takes six, seven or ten, perhaps even fourteen days from the moment of infection before the transformation of the entire internal organism into psora has been effected. Then only, there follows after a slight or more severe chill in the evening and a general heat, followed by perspiration in the following night, [a little fever which by many persons is ascribed to a cold and therefore disregarded], the outbreak of the vesicles of itch, at first fine as if from miliary fever, but afterwards enlarging on the skin, first in the region of the spot first infected, and, indeed, accompanied with a voluptuously tickling itching which may be called unbearably agreeable, which compels the patient so irresistibly to rub and to scratch the vesicles of itch, that, if a person restrains himself forcibly from rubbing or scratching, a shudder passes over the skin of the whole body.

This rubbing and scratching indeed satisfies somewhat for a few moments, but there then follows immediately a long continued burning of the part affected. Late in the evening and before midnight this itching is most frequent and most unbearable.

Far from being an independent, merely local, cutaneous disease, the vesicles or pustules of itch are the reliable proof that the completion of the internal Psora has already been effected, and the eruption is merely an integrating factor of the same; for this peculiar eruption and this peculiar itching make a part of the essence of the whole disease in its natural, least dangerous state.

Only this skin symptom of the psora which has permeated the whole organism, only this eruption, as well as the sores which later arise from it and are attended on their borders with the itching peculiar to psora, as also the herpes which has this peculiar itching and which becomes humid when rubbed [the tetter], as also the Tinea capitis-these alone can propagate this disease to other persons, because they alone contain the communicable miasma of the psora.

- But the remaining secondary symptoms of the psora, which in time manifest themselves after the disappearance or the artificial expulsion of the eruption, i.e., the general psoric ailments, cannot at all communicate this disease to others. They are, so far as we know, just as little able to transfer the psora to others, as the secondary symptoms of the venereal disease are able to infect other men as observed with syphilis.

In this state, the disease is most easily cured through specific remedies internally administered.

But if the disease is allowed to advance in its peculiar course without the use of an internal curative remedy or an external application to drive away the eruption, the whole disease within rapidly increases, and this increase of the internal malady makes necessary a corresponding increase of the skin-symptom. The itch-eruption, therefore, in order to be able to soothe and to keep latent the increased internal malady, has to spread and must finally cover the whole surface of the body.

Yet even at this juncture of the disease the patient still appears healthy in every other respect; all the symptoms of the internal Psora, now so much increased, still remain covered through the skin-symptom augmented in the same proportion. But so great a torture, as is caused by so unbearable an itching spread over the whole body, even the most robust man cannot continue to bear. He endeavors to free himself from these torments at any price, and, as there is no thorough help for him with the physicians of the old school, he endeavors to secure deliverance at least from this eruption, which itches so unbearably, even if it should cost his life; and the means are soon furnished him, either by other ignorant persons, or by Allopathic physicians and surgeons. He seeks deliverance from his external tortures, without suspecting the greater misfortune that unavoidably follows, and is bound to follow, on the expulsion of the external skin-symptom.

But the ignorance of the uninstructed layman may be pardoned if he drives out the itch-eruption and the troublesome itching by a cold shower-bath, for he does not know to what dangerous accidents and outbreaks of the Psora-disease, that lurks within, he thereby opens the door.

Even when the itch-disease has reached this high degree, the eruption, together with the internal malady, in one word, the whole Psora, may still be healed by the internal, specific homoeopathic remedies, with greater difficulty, indeed, than in the beginning, immediately after its origin, but still far more easily and certainly than after a complete expulsion of the eruption by mere external applications, when we must cure the internal psora as it brings forth its secondary symptoms and develops into nameless chronic diseases.

Chapter 3

Why Hahnemann Thought of Miasma[2,13,9,25]

We would try to trace the history of the theory of miasma and the reasons why Hahnemann thought it is necessary to think miasmatically in treatment of chronic diseases.

"The internal essential nature of every malady, of every individual case of disease (as far as it is necessary for us to know it for the purpose of curing it) expresses itself by the symptoms, as they present themselves to the investigations of the true observer in their extent, connection and succession."

"When the physician has discovered all the observable symptoms of the disease that exist, he has discovered the disease itself, he has attained the complete conception of it requisite to enable to effect a cure."

The same doctrine is written in § 6 of The Organon.

"The unprejudiced observer, takes note of nothing in every individual disease except the changes in the health of the body and of the mind which can be perceived externally by means of the sense, that is to say, he notices only the deviations from the former healthy state of the now diseased individual. All these perceptible signs represent the disease in its whole extent that is together they form the true and only conceivable portrait of the disease."

In the footnote of § 6 he ridiculous those who would seek to know anything more about the disease than the symptoms presented by the patient, After all this we would hardly expect to meet Hahnemann in the domain of pathological hypothesis and actually propagating a theory of the origin of all chronic diseases based on actual pathogens of itch, figwart disease, Chancre.

What happened? What was Hahnemann trying to do?

Hahnemann was actually looking for a deeply seated fundamental malady, whose parts were manifested by the new symptoms that appeared from time to time. Unless he knew the fundamental disease in its full extent and knew all the symptoms peculiar to it, he could not hope to discover any medicines which should correspond in their effects to the whole fundamental malady and therefore he would be unable to cure it in its whole extent.

To know what was in Hahnemann's mind let's read § 103:

"The miasmatic chronic maladies, which, I have shown, always remain the same in their essential nature, especially the psora, must be in investigated, as to the whole sphere of their symptoms, in a much more minute manner than has ever been done before, for in them also one patient only exhibits a portion of their symptoms, a second, a third and so on, present some other symptoms. Which constitute the entire extent of this chronic malady, so that the whole array of the symptoms belonging to such a miasmatic, chronic disease can only be ascertained from the observation of very many individual patients affected with such a chronic disease."

Thus it is clear that Hahnemann set out to define a picture of true chronic diseases in its complete extent in human race. A kind of collective disease, a part of which is expressed in an individual at a given point of time.

And why did he want to do it? The answer is given in § 103:

"Without a complete survey and collective picture of these symptoms the medicines capable of curing the whole malady homoeopathically cannot be discovered. These remedies are at the same time the true remedies of the several patients suffering from such chronic affections."

Miasma means, taint, stain or pollute. Now Hahnemann chose this word because he thought that there must be a fundamental pollution in the vital force.

"Miasma are fundamental diseases and everyone who manifest the disease (in whatever form or name) has the same disease which is expressed to us by unique set of symptoms based on the individual constitution, temperament and environment of an individual."

Hahnemann compares acute miasms with the uniquely occurring epidemic disease in § 100, in which he states that each reigning epidemic is in many regards a phenomenon of a particular kind that is found to deviate greatly from all former epidemics.

"This is true of all contagious diseases except those that stem form an invariable infectious tinder, such as smallpox, measles etc."

Hahnemann compares the chronic miasm with the uniquely occurring collective diseases in § 103, in which he states,

"Just like the mostly acute epidemics, the chronic wasting sickness remains the same as to their dynamis. Just as I did with epidemics, I had to investigate the chronic wasting sickness (namely and principally psora) much more exactly than ever before. I had to do this because of the extent of the symptoms in these chronic diseases and also because one patient carries only a part of the symptoms in himself, while a second or third patient suffers from some other bafflement which as it were are only a part torn off from the totality of the symptoms that make up the entire extent of the one and the same disease. Therefore, the complex of all the symptoms belonging to such a miasmatic wasting sickness (in particular, psora) can only be ascertained from very many such individual chronic patients, without such a complete overview and total image, the medicines that are homoeopathically curative for the whole wasting sickness cannot be searched out."

In the chronic disease Hahnemann states "thousands of tedious ailments of humanity are the true descendents of many-formed Psora alone; they are merely descendents of one and the same vast original malady."

In § 81, Hahnemann remarks that it is "understandable how Psora could now unfold itself in so many countless disease forms in all the human race since this age old infectious tinder has gone, little by little, through many milestones of human organisms over the course of hundred of generations, thus attaining an incredible proliferation."

This suggests that Psora has various characteristic embodiments over time but the disease dynamis remains the same.

In the chronic disease (Pg. No. 10-12) Hahnemann indicates that some such mutations have taken place with regards to the manifestation of Psora.

He indicates that Psora began primarily as an itching eruption of the skin. It then manifested primarily as Leprosy, which was a further development of this skin condition, and was still characterized by a violent itch, it later (with suppression) became less of a skin condition and more an internal itch diathesis with secondary manifestation of great variety.

Hahnemann first conceived his doctrine of chronic diseases about the year 1827, he says that from the year 1816-17 the solution of this problem occupied him day and night then he summoned his two closest disciples, Dr. Stapf and Dr. Gross and his book was published in the following year, changing the face of homoeopathy forever.

The comparative study of the first four successive editions of Organon (1810-1819-1824-1829) especially the sections 39-61 shows that Hahnemann was all the time struggling hard to reduce to order the vast chaotic mass of facts concerning diseases. He weighed every sort of classification of diseases in the balance and found each of them wanting.

His realistic mind was always for concrete individual cases and abhorred abstractions which the nosological studies of diseases afforded in his time. He came to the conclusion: "Nature has no nomenclature or classification of diseases. She produces single diseases etc." (Vie Sec. 46 of the 1st edition of Organon and retained right up to the 3rd edition of Organon.) But about some diseases he was not so sure as they were so fixed in their character and course. They might have been caused by a peculiar contagion (a peculiar miasm of tolerably fixed character) e.g. Plague, Small-pox etc.: so that each of them can be given a peculiar name.

Though we find Hahnemann constantly busy in developing the knowledge of drugs and perfecting the art of therapeutics, there was no time when his mind was not occupied with the knowledge of diseases and how to improve it. That is why the main changes in the successive editions of Organon deal with nannies of conceptions about the vital force and about the causative factors of diseases. In the first three editions of Organon we come across the term "miasm" but it was used in the accepted sense of that era and its precise connotation and denotation had not yet been fixed by Hahnemann. During Hahnemann's time all the morbific agents were designated by a general term "miasm or miasma"-which literally meant "any noxious emanation or effluvia or a polluting factor." There was no fixed connotation or denotation attached to the term "miasm."

Hahnemann was the first to perceive and teach the parasitical nature of contagious diseases e.g., small-pox, Chicken-pox, Measles, Scarlet fever, etc. i.e., most of the acute diseases of epidemic and sporadic character depended upon a "contagium vivum," Though he made it explicit in his article on cholera in 1831 ("An Appeal to the thinking philanthropists respecting the mode of propagation of the Asiatic Cholera" Coethen, October 24th, 1831) he must have arrived at it before 1827 when he expressed his views on Chronic Diseases to his two disciples before publishing his book on 'Chronic Diseases' in 1828. If we read between the lines of 'Chronic Diseases' in is evident even to a casual reader how he based his arguments on the notion of acute miasms which he had arrived at previously. He arrived at the final conclusion about the nature of miasmatic conception through there steps of thinking:

1. First he came to a definite idea about the biological agents being causally related to acute diseases
2. Secondly, he was able to show the analogy between the mode of onset and development of acute as well as chronic diseases; and
3. Thirdly, he established the contagious nature of Chronic Diseases during one phase of their development in the human organism.
4. The possibility of transmission of those disease factors through successive generations was established through Hahnemann's marvelous collections of facts from the earliest possible recorded history.

So from all these observations he could assert the causative factors of chronic diseases as being of miasmatic nature with the same conception of miasm which he attached in relation to acute diseases. That is why after much deliberations and prolonged observation Hahnemann added the following line in section 72 of Organon, 5th edition: they (i.e., chronic diseases) are caused by dynamic infection with a miasm.

Chapter 4

Why Should We Know Miasma[2]

Hering in his introductory remarks in the Organon (3rd American edition) thought that it is not of vital importance to know misama: "what important influence can it exert whether a homoeopath adopt the theoretical opinion of Hahnemann or not, so long as he holds the principal tools of the master and the Materia Medica of our schools? What influence can it have, whether a physician adopts or rejects the Psoric theory as long as he always selects the most similar medicine possible?"

Allen gives an apt reply:

The last line is well timed "so long as he selects the most similar medicine possible". The fact is, we cannot select the most similar remedy possible until we understand the phenomena of the active and latent miasm; for the true similia is always based upon the existing basic miasm, whether we be conscious or unconscious of the fact.

We should know, not only the name of that underlying principle that fathers the phenomena with which we are so diligently contending and combating. It is the difference between an intelligent warfare and fighting in the dark.

Suppose we prescribe the similar remedy and have no knowledge of the laws of action and reaction (or primary or secondary reaction), how can we watch the progress of a case without a definite knowledge of these disease forces (miasm), with their mysterious but persistent, progressions, pauses, rests, forward movements, retreats and attacks along unfamiliar lines, and whose multiplied mode of action we have taken no cognizance? In fact, if we know nothing about the traits and characteristics of miasma, is it possible to wage an equal warfare?

Knowledge of all miasmatic phenomena would be, in toto, a complete knowledge of all that is known as disease, and beyond these symptoms there is nothing discoverable or recognizable as disease.

In our study of miasmatics, we are brought into a closer relation with the nature and cause of the disease. Indeed the diseases become no longer a mystery, but a clear problem, which is to be solved by a careful study of the phenomena that each case presents; each case being a distinct and separate study in itself.

Our cures are not made through the application of our therapeutics to a nomenclature, but to a classical grouping of all the phenomena therein presented and that which we see is often not seen by the physician who has no knowledge of the miasmatics.

If we fail to understand the miasmatic phenomena, and the relation they bear to each other, and also to the life force, we fail to select the true basic remedy.

In order to arrest pathological developments or processes we must search for the basic miasmatic symptoms in each case. Because even after we have dispelled the effects of acute diseases by our apsoric remedies, the psoric or chronic miasmatic process has been forced to set up a stasis or a new central point of elimination for its own pathologic debris.

In sequel to acute disease this of course becomes unnecessary if we take into consideration the chronic miasmatic process that was co-operative with the acute disease. Then we not only arrest he whole process but we also shorten the disease period and the suffering of our patients.

In cases that do not yield to treatment, even homoeopathic we must always be lookout for the basic miasm.

If we have some understanding of the nature of the miasms, their history and action upon the life of the organism, we are able to follow these processes, linking them together into an unbroken chain, and our knowledge is not confined to the present, but it becomes prophetic and we can give a possible prognosis of developments in our patients.

RELEVANCE OF MIASM THEORY IN CLINICAL PRACTICE[5]

Miasms go beyond the infectious diseases they are associated with. They indicate a greater pattern, giving a more complete picture of the nature of the disease and the prognosis. Recognising miasmatic patterns in a person's disease process will aid in the search for the similimum. Just like a person, remedies also have miasmatic traits. Often the remedies will display the features of more than one miasm with a clear center in one, for example, *Calcarea carbonica*, which is considered as a great antipsoric, has strong sycotic features such as glandular swelling and induration, tendency to obesity, and genital cysts. Through careful study of the Materia Medica we can see these reaction patterns in all of our remedies and can see the affinities of certain remedies to particular disease states. Incorporating the miasmatic patterns in the person and their illness and matching this to the remedy will increase the chances of finding the similimum.

KENT ON WHY MUST WE KNOW THE MIASMA?[20,21]

Manifestly it is a good thing to know the history of a patient, all the peculiarities of the life of the patient. It is important to know whether the patient is syphilitic or sycotic. You know that everybody is Psoric but those who have lived a proper life have escaped the two contagious diseases, which man acquires on the first place by his own seeking.

If a patient has gone to the end of typhoid or some lingering disease, you know that he is psoric. But if you also know that he is syphilitic or sycotic you can conduct his convalescence into a speedy recovery. If he denies these things you may be puzzled. The sycotic patient may go into a state of do-nothing and decline at the end of a typhoid fever. Convalescence will not be established. He will lie with aversion to food. He does not react. He does not repair. There is no tissue regeneration, no assimilation. There is no vitality he lays in a semi-quiescent state; there is no convalescing in the matter. If you know he is a sycotic patient he must have an anti-sycotic remedy, and then he will begin to rally. If such a patient is syphilitic, he must have an anti-syphilitic remedy. If neither of this miasma is present a remedy looking towards his Psoric state will cause him to rally.

The nature of these cases must be kept in view. Remember these chronic miasma are present in the internal state and after an acute illness very often have to be fought. If this is not known, many patients will gradually sink and die for apparent want of vitality to convalescence.

The susceptibility is laid by his inheritance, just as our parents lay the susceptibility to Psora and syphilis. Man can only have one attack of one of the three chronic miasmas in his natural lifetime. A man can not take syphilis twice, he can not take sycosis twice and can not take Psora twice. One attack alters immunity of that person forever.

The more the human race becomes susceptible to all the miasmas the more they become complicated with each other the more the human race becomes susceptible to acute and epidemic diseases.

SECTION II: THEORY OF MIASMA AFTER HANNEMANN

Chapter: 5
Hahnemann, Samuel

Chapter: 6
Allen, J.H.

Chapter: 7
Kent, James Taylor

Chapter: 8
Roberts, H.A.

Chapter: 9
Paschero, T.P.

Chapter: 10
Eizayaga and Ortega

Chapter: 11

Julian, O.A.

Chapter: 12

H. Mantfort, Cabello

Chapter: 13

Sankaran, Rajan

Chapter: 14

Nigam, Harsh

Chapter: 15

Current understanding of miasma

Chapter 5

Hahnemann, Samuel[15,16,9]

In the course of his clinical work, Hahnemann noticed that there were certain chronic conditions that he could not treat satisfactorily with homoeopathy. He searched for an explanation of why certain persons were not cured after repetition of the similimum. He noticed, in some cases, that after each dose of a well-chosen remedy, there was less and less of a response.

He concluded that it was not due to a failure of the method but that he had not solved the question of the chronic diseases. Hahnemann wrote that this question constantly occupied his mind for 12 years from 1816 to 1828. The results of his thinking were contained in a major treatise, Chronic Diseases, which he wrote from 1828 to 1830, and developed further in the second edition written between 1835 and 1839. Chronic Diseases consists of five volumes, the first being purely theoretical in which Hahnemann outlines his miasm theory and its relevance for the treatment of chronic disease. The remaining four volumes are practical and contain detailed descriptions of a number of remedy pictures.

Hahnemann's Three Basic Chronic Miasms The word 'miasm' comes from the Greek word meaning polluting or staining. Miasmatic theory was one of the theories for the cause of disease, prevailing in the 18th and 19th century. At the time Hahnemann formulated his theory there was no knowledge of infection in microbiological terms.

Hahnemann postulated that there were three distinct miasms: syphilis, sycosis and psora. Syphilis was a condition which was clearly identified as contagious, even in Hahnemann's own time and in using these labels for his miasmatic traits, Hahnemann clearly implied that chronic disease has its genesis in contagion, or person to person transmission. Moreover, by applying rational theory to the manifestations, which we now attribute to different stages of infection, Hahnemann reasoned that the miasmatic Influence eventually affects the whole organism, ultimately giving rise to a skin eruption after the miasm has penetrated the entire body. He associated each of the three miasms with characteristic skin manifestations:

- Psora - Eruption (vesicle, tetter, tinea)
- Sycosis - figwart
- Syphilis Chancer

Hahnemann believed Psora to be the main cause of chronic diseases, making up seven-eighths of the total incidence, with one-eighth being caused by the sexually transmitted Sycosis and Syphilis. He considered psora to be the oldest miasm, dating back to antiquity where it manifested itself as scabies. During the middle Ages he postulated that it became more aggressive in the form of leprosy, becoming milder again to present as scabies in modern times. The Hebrew word tsorat meaning a groove, fault, or stigma, was a term often applied to lepers and to those affected during the great plagues, and conveys what Hahnemann had in mind.

Complicating this model was a combination of one or two miasms, which made treatment very difficult and rendered certain cases incurable.

He considered that these miasmatic conditions were curable only as long as the local reactions were still present. Alternatively, progress could be achieved if skin eruptions could be evoked again in the course of treatment.

In Organon Hahnemann suggests that Miasma lurk inside body and can be activated by several of factors to derange health in a particular form of chronic disease.

This was a simple but a brilliant working model considering the era of scientific darkness he lived in.

PSORA

Tsorat; Hebrew = groove, fault, stigmata

The hydra headed monster

The fundamental cause of all chronic disease

The main presentation ITCH + Eruption

SYCOSIS

Associated with Gonorrhoea

The main presentation = CONDYLOMATA + Gleet

SYPHILIS

Associated with syphilis

The main presentation = ULCER + bubo

Table 1: Hahnemann's Three Basic Chronic Miasms

Miasma	Psora	Sycosis	Syphilis
Cutaneous presentation	Itch, Eruption, Herpes and Tatter	Condylomata, Gleet	Ulcer, Bubo

Chapter 6

Allen, J.H.[2]

1. Allen proposed Psoric Theory of Disease

    (a) Hahnemann states that the fundamental cause of all disease (including Sycosis & Syphilis) is Psora. Actually what Hahnemann is propagating as his theory of causation of chronic miasmatic diseases is what Allen refers to as the psoric theory of disease.

    (b) Hahnemann's hypothesis was that chronic disease are chronic because some unknown devitalizing principal subverts life forces in such a way that the dynamic mistunement of health cannot be corrected. He called these unknown devitalizing principles to be chronic miasma (miasma = emanation spreading in the air exerting a morbid influence).

    (c) This was Hahnemann's theory while medical science accepted another theory at that time that is Virchow's cellular pathology theory. Virchow's cell, the unit of life was vivified, by chemical processes or by chemical changes. At that very time Koch formulated the germ theory of disease.

(d) For Hahnemann and Homoeopathy the guiding fundamental principles are-the dynamic origin of disease, the dynamization of drug & the application of similia.

2. Allen proposed Bond of Psora with Life Forces

   (a) In the study of Psoric theory of disease we must not look from the bio-chemical side, but from Vital/ Potential side (Bio-physical side).

   (b) Psora is that potential which when becomes well bonded with the life force, it cooperates with this life force. Together these two along with other miasms, cause all physiological deflections, functional disturbances followed by structural and pathological changes.

   (c) Under the influence of perverted life action psora' life force is no longer a true dynamis but it is in bond with another dynamis, psora which knows no law and has no life giving qualities in it in fact all the dealings of psora are destructive.

   (d) It is the same with miasmatic potential; it is an invisible and unseen thing, yet we see the effects of its presence in the organism long before any changes of tissue take place. We see it first as a rule, first manifest in the mental sphere, then in the physiological or functional, then, finally, in the pathological. The pathological, of course, coming last.

3. Allen proposed Potential Study of Miasmatics

   (a) We generally see the landmarks of one of these chronic miasms stamped upon the organism. We see it in every feature and every physiological process; in the shape and contour of the body; upon the visual expression; we see it on the skin; by the response in the very inner being, the mental, the moral, even the spiritual, give us responses of the presence and influence of miasm.

(b) We see disease to be expression of three basic potential (patho-physiological trends). He who has become acquainted with the higher homoeopathics of Hahnemann, which comprises not only of disease potentials, but the drug action, can apply the law of similia at a deeper level.

(c) As we study these miasm, we see they express themselves in their degrees of action (primary secondary and tertiary); and in their nature (acute, chronic and latent).

4. Allen proposed Pseudo Psora for the first time. Allen observed a new miasma which he named Pseudo Psora which latter came to be known as Tubercular miasma.

Chapter 7

Kent, James Tyler[20,21]

James Tyler Kent introduced metaphysical ideas into miasm theory, which stem from his Swedenborgian background. Like Hahnemann he attributed the cause of all disease to psora. According to Kent, however, it is never possible for psora to manifest itself in a healthy race; a weakness must be there first.

He considered this weakness to be original sin, a legacy passed from generation to generation. The syphilitic and sycotic miasms can be contracted through sexual contact, not so psora.

Kent interprets psora as a product of impure thought and human materialism which is itself the precursor of physical degeneration. Kent correlates the diseases of humankind to their aspirations which he interprets as the mirror of their innermost parts.

Kent was also amongst the first to interpret the pathological aspect of miasma.

The primary skin reaction in psora consists of vesicular eruptions. The concept of all pervading miasm suggested to Kent that it is physically seated in the circulatory vasculature.

The mucocutaneous manifestations associated with syphilis are, firstly, the chancre and secondly, the bubo. By this reasoning, tissue destruction is a key characteristic associated with both the disease and its miasmatic counterparts. The proposed loci for the syphilitic miasm are periosteum, bones and brain, as would be expected from the tissue pathologies associated with secondary and tertiary syphilis.

Kent observed an affinity of the sycotic miasm to the soft tissues and those stemming from the mesoderm. He described the sycotic taint as waxy with pale lips, translucent ears, with warts and papillomata. Mucous membranes such as the conjunctiva and sinuses are usually affected. Children born with sycotic tendencies are of a waxy anaemic complexion, they have a poor digestion, their stools frequently contain undigested food, they are worse for heat and fail to thrive. Hahnemann had a very limited understanding of sycosis. Kent took Hahnemann's ideas further, empirically researching the pattern of sycosis. He gives a useful description of his observations in his lecture notes on Materia Medica in the chapter *Natrium sulphuricum* and sycosis.

Following Kent's argument to its logical conclusion, many conditions can be conceptually linked to one of the miasms in terms of their tissue involvement and pathology.

Table 2: Miasms and Pathology

Miasma	Tissue	Pathology	Result
Psora	Cutaneous tissue	Inflammation	Desquamation
Sycosis	Mesodermal and Endothelial	Proliferation	Fungation
Syphilis	Submucosal and Periosteal	Destruction	Induration / caseation

Chapter 8

Roberts, H.A.[28]

H A Roberts linked the miasmatic stigmata with disturbed assimilation. Whereas psora has difficulty in assimilating constructive elements the sycotic patient tends to assimilate to the point of over-growth.

He considered psora to be a deficiency state. Functional disturbances manifest themselves due to lack of vital elements in the system or the inability to assimilate them from foods. There are no structural changes associated with psora; in his definition these occur in combination with the other miasms. Symptoms are closely related to emotional disturbances. Roberts described the mental condition as one of the strongest characteristics of latent psora. These patients are mentally alert, their mind is keen, anxiety states dominate. There is also restlessness (physical & mental itch).

Roberts expands on the picture of sycosis by painting a mental image. He describes the sycotic patient as being exceedingly suspicious, not even trusting her/himself. As a result this person goes back to do or say things over again. The sycotic person has the suspicion they will not be fully understood and others will give the wrong meaning to what she/he conveys. This suspicion can lead to jealousy. The most degenerate features of the sycotic nature are the suspicion, the tendency to harm others and themselves and animals. Quarrelsomeness and irritability are also displayed in the sycotic psychology. The syphilitic state is characterised by structural changes. There are far fewer sensitivities to environment and food. Overall there are also fewer subjective symptoms. The syphilitic appearance is characterized by a large head, moist, gluey, greasy hair with an offensive odour, hair falling out in bunches. Syphilis is known to deform everything. Ulcerations are the mark of the syphilitic stigmata.

Table 3: Miasms and characteristics of metabolism and tissue reaction according to Roberts

Miasma	Keyword	Characteristics of metabolism	Tissue reaction	Mention
Psora	Deficiency	Under assimilation outward loss	Structure intact	Anxiety neurosis
Sycosis	Excess	Over assimilation Inward retentiveness	Overgrowth	Obsessive states
Syphilis	Disorganised	Self assimilation inner and outer disruption	Deformity	Psychosis

Chapter 9

Paschero, T.P.[27,1,46,47]

Paschero defines psora as a morbid derangement of the whole body imprinted on genome, a particular reactional mode against pathogenic agents.

Psoric defensive reaction = Supernormal or Hyperergic Response limited to functional states with no structural or gross pathology. He identifies the neurovegetative as the mediator of psoric response and he concludes: that there is no difference between psora and allergy, apart from clinical expression Ortega describes three forms of cellular functional alteration, which he relates to the three chronic miasms:

Defect = psora

Excess = sycosis

Perversion = syphilis

Chapter 10

Eizayaga[26,18,24] and Ortega

Eizayaga relates the miasms to disturbances of the most important vital functions:

Excitation = psora

Dysfunction = sycosis

Inhibition = syphilis

Psora is the state of hyper excitation of vital functions, a dynamic lack of balance of the vital force. It is associated with functional, not lesional disturbances.

He sees sycosis as perverted functional activity, leading to hypertrophy of the ego and tissues - perversion of feelings, especially those related to love. Thus the sycotic taint is associated with sexual perversion, obsession, reservation, suspicion, aggressiveness, jealousy.

Chapter 11

Julian, O.A.[19]

In 1984, O. A. Julian and M. Haffen give a view of miasms, based in modern concepts of genetics, biochemistry, molecular biology, toxicology, immunology and ecology. Briefly:

1. **Psora is renamed as 'Dysimmunosis'** = Altered immunologic response. The multiple aetiologic agents include: aggression of mineral, chemical, vegetable and animal origins. Psora has multiple manifestations including 'metastatis and morbid alternate faces'.

2. **Syphilis** = is renamed as **'Dysmorphogenosis'**. The inherited and damaged information is transmitted in an autosomic dominant pattern.

3. **Sycosis = is renamed 'Dysmetabolosis'**.

    It is based in defects in two areas:

    • Enzymes-catabolic pathways.
    • Transport across cellular membranes.

    Both conditions have a base in damaged and mutated DNA.

Chapter 12

H. Montfort-Cabello[42]

If we review the normal and abnormal repair mechanism of cells and tissues, the classic concept of miasma as obstacles to Vital force trying to cure a diseased organism does not seem to be appropriate. Instead of being considered as obstacles in healing procedure, we should see them, as inherited or acquired, disturbed repair mechanisms of cells and tissues or 'dysrepair'.

Linking these types of 'dysrepair' with knowledge of the homoeopathic concept of reactional modes give the following results:

1. The psoric reactional mode can be understood as a defect in molecular repair (e.g., asthma, epilepsy and high blood pressure).
2. The syphilitic reactional mode can be understood as a defect in the apoptotic process, which leads cells to an anticipated death (e.g., Alzheimer) or to necrosis, producing ulcerative and destructive lesions (e.g., ulcerative colitis).
3. The sycosis reactional mode can be understood as a defect in control of cell division and extracellular matrix production, due to mutation in DNA repair consequences and excessive cell and ECM proliferation with tumor production and fibrous tissue formation.

Chapter 13

Sankaran, Rajan[29]

Sankaran introduces the interesting idea of linking the three chronic miasms to stages in our lives.

He considers that youth is susceptible to acute miasms. Responses at this time are quick and illness can be easily thrown off. The threats are external and provoke a strong instinctive reaction.

During early adulthood there is still much energy, liveliness and activity (psora) and an openness to express fear and anxiety. Then there comes a struggle to succeed. There is hope and failure does not mean the end of the world.

Then middle age sets in (sycosis). We realize our limitations and to preserve face we start to cover up: hiding our incapacities in order to be accepted. Our reactions and habits are more fixed. This might be seen by some as true for our society. Wisdom and age are no longer valued. People are seen as resources and have a place as long as they keep up with the set pace. The elderly feel they are no longer valued so they try to hide this for as long as possible.

Then comes old age (syphilitic). The time for letting go and decay. This is reflected in the syphilitic miasm. There is despair about recovery but unlike psora without hope.

Chapter 14

Nigam, Harsh[25,50]

Recognizes Miasma as dynamic alteration of dynamic vital force, and he recognizes that stamp of miasma is visible at every level of the human organism including mind, autonomic nervous system, metabolic processes, reproductive, repair, Anabolic processes, Catabolic and apoptotic processes, hormonal and autoregulatory mechanisms and on the even human form. Since Hahnemann's time pathophysiology has moved on and now one thing is clear that in the genesis of disease, immunity is the common denominator. It is clear now that chronic diseases as well as acute diseases are caused by disordered immunity. Even the mental diseases ruin health via immunity. This has been established by psycho-neuro-immunology

We can explore miasma theory on the basis of immunity. This author has tried to do so.

Immunity and Homoeopathy

i. Altered immunity ⟶ Hypersensitivity reaction ⟶ Immuno damage ⟶ Chronic disease

ii. Immunodeficiency state ⟶ external pathogens cause direct cellular damage ⟶ Chronic disease. Please take note that Psoric reactional mode is an oscillatory reactional mode because it oscillates between Hypersensitivity reactional immuno-state and Hypo-immuno reactional states.

iii. By this logic Hypersensitivity immuno reactions are fundamentally Psoric reactional mode (Psora is the fundamental cause of all diseases-Hahnemann)

iv. Immuno damage caused by hypersensitivity leads to a spectrum of disorders there are five types of basic hypersensitivity reaction discussed further in section III.

v. The author draws similarity of five miasmas to five basic hypersensitivity reaction in the table below:

Table 4: Hypersensitivity Tissue Damage & Miasma

Type I	IgE Mediated Hypersensitivity	Anaphylaxis	Psoric [Itch]
Type II	Complement Mediated Hypersensitivity	Cytotoxic Reaction	Syphilitic [Cell destruction]
Type III	Igm, IgG Mediated Hypersensitivity	Arthus Reaction	Sycotic [Thrombus Formation]
Type IV	T-Cell Mediated Hypersensitivity	CMI Delayed Hypersensitivity	Tubercular [Granuloma Formation]
Type V	Ag-Ab Mediated Hypersensitivity	Stimulatory Type	Cancer [Stimulate]

Chapter 15

Current Understanding of Miasma

We must now draw these concepts together (physical, metabolic, histological, pathological, reactive, psychological and immunological) The miasmatic pictures that emerge from this data are rather like the conjoint remedy pictures that are assembled from desperate proving symptoms of a remedy. Some homoeopathic physicians find such conceptual groupings useful in coming to a prescription, since they narrow the field of search and provide a conceptual base.

The recognition of a predominant miasm, insofar as such a thing exists, can be something of a lifeline to a prescriber who is struggling with a multitude of imponderables and indefinite prescribing data. The speculative and subjective aspects of miasm theory, however, make it a guide rather than a maxim.

In the intervening years since Hahnemann described the three chronic miasms, further miasms (intercalated miasms) have been recognised. H.C. Allen proposed the concept of mixed miasm and defined two:

Psora + Syphilis = phthisis

Psora + Sycosis = Scrofula.

The French homoeopaths first recognized Cancer as a separate miasm Psora + Sycosis + Syphilis = Cancer

Universally modern homoeopaths now recognize five Miasma: Psora, Sycosis, Syphilis, Tubercular and Cancer. Here first three are basic or simple miasm while last two are mixed or complicated miasm.

SECTION III: IMMUNITY & MIASMA

Chapter 16
Concepts of Immune system

Chapter 17
Concept of immunologic balance

Chapter 18
Immunity & diseases

Chapter 19
Immunity & Homoeopathy

Chapter 16

Concepts of Immune System[36,33,50]

I. INTRODUCTION

Von Pirquet (1909) put forward an hypothesis to explain the versatility & complexity of the immune response. He coined the term "allergy" to mean changed reactivity. One change he recognized as Immunity and the other as Hypersensitivity. Von Pirquet made no distinction between the beneficial & the harmful expression of the immune response & suggested they were all manifestations of a common biologic process of sensitization which he encompassed by the term allergy. As irony would have it, today words of Von Pirquet are used differently.

Over the years the term immunity has come to mean that which Pirquet defined as allergy, and allergy has come to mean as hypersensitivity.

II. OVERVIEW OF IMMUNE SYSTEM

- Immunity is defined as an ability of the organism to resist foreign material

Concepts of Immune System

- Homoeopathically speaking, Immunity is a mechanism by which the vital force destroys or resists foreign material

III. CLASSIFICATION OF IMMUNITY

A. Innate Immunity
B. Acquired/Adaptive Immunity
    1. NON-SPECIFIC IMMUNITY
    2 SPECIFIC IMMUNITY
        a. HUMORAL IMMUNITY
        b. CMI (Cell Mediated Immunity)

IV. EFFECTOR CELLS INVOLVED IN IMMUNE RESPONSE

Effector Cells Involved in Immune response are blood Cells (WBC's) which are:

(A) SARC (Special Antigen Regulator Cell) or Lymphoid cells:
    a. T - Lymphocyte or T Cells
    b. B - Lymphocyte or B Cells
    c. Natural Killer Cells or NK Cells
    d. Marrow dependent Cells or M Cells

(B) Mediator Cells
    i Neutrophil or Polymorphoneuclear leukocytes (PMN)
    ii. Monocyte - Macrophage
    iii. Basophil – Mast Cells
    iv. Eosinophil

SARC (SPECIAL ANTIGEN REGULATOR CELL)

- Lymphocytic system provides cells of the specific immune system.
- These cells react to the antigen in an specific way. These are lymphoid cells.
- **B Cells** are produced in Bone Marrow (B stands for Bursa of fabricius which is site of B Cells production in birds) B Cells are responsible for Humoral Immunity.
- **T Cells** are produced in thymus during embryonic development and responsible for CMI. T cells are of two types CD4 + or Helper T Cells which increase Immunoglobulin production by B Cell i.e. Help B Cell. CD8 + T cells or Cytotoxic T cell or killer, K Cells.
- **N K Cells** destroy malignant cells & virus laiden cells.
- **M Cells** are responsible for rejection of graft and destruction of oncogenic virus.

MEDIATOR CELLS & MEDIATOR

- Cells which contain substances having biologic properties which can amplify the effects of phagocytosis called as Mediator cells
- Chemical in Mediator cells is called as Mediator
- Mediators cause Increased vascular permeability & amplification of inflammation

Neutrophils are mature circulating cells that destroy bacteria/ viruses by engulfing them, i.e. by phagocytosis. **Monocytes** are immature circulating cells which when fixed in tissues are cells as macrophage which are more powerful phagocytic agent than neutrophils. **Basophils** are circulating cells which when fixed in tissues are converted into mast cells which contain Heparin whose function is to prevent coagulation of blood, they also release Histamine/

Bradykinin/SRS-A/Serotonin which are chemical mediators of inflammation which cause Anaphylaxis or Hyper Sensitivity Reaction.

Eosinophil has a function to detoxify foreign protein therefore they increase in worm infestation. Eosinophil collect at the site of Antigen-Antibody reaction and phagocytose these immune complexes and therefore are greatly increased in Allergic phenomenon. In inflammation Eosinophil remove Histamine/Bradykinin/Serotonin and other products of inflammation to limit or 'wall off' inflammation.

V. FOREIGNNESS

- The immune response is impartial in its dealings with foreignness
- It rejects whatever it recognizes as non self, ranging from pollen to transplanted organ
- Foreignness in language of immunity is called as an Antigen.

A. WHAT IS AN ANTIGEN?

- Any substance that fulfils the following criteria is classified as an antigen:
    a. Non self
    b. Molecular weight. Of more than 10,000 D
    c. Stereochemical structure.
    d. Haptanes.

B. TACKLING FOREIGNNESS

- Immune mediated destruction has five components of host's encounter with foreignness
    1. ENVIRONMENT
    2. TARGET CELL
    3. PHAGOCYTIC CELL

4. MEDIATOR CELL
5. SARC (Special Antigen Regulator Cell)

C. ENVIRONMENT

- Foreign substances which have the capacity to evoke immunologic response are referred to as ANTIGEN.
- ALLERGENS are a specialized class of antigen that take part in Humoral or CMI type hypersensitivity response.

D. PORTAL OF ENTRY OF AN ANTIGEN

- Ingestion
- Inhalation
- Contact
- Injection

VI. TARGET CELL

- Target Cells are cells upon which the environmental AGENT has an impact
- These can be: SKIN/GIT/RESP/CIRCULATORY/RENAL etc.
- The effect of AGENT will vary according to the type & location of the Target cell. e.g. Respiratory tact, Bronchospasm etc.
- CVS → Endothelial target → Edema & injury to target cell
- Injury to Target Cell can be direct or Indirect
- Indirect Injury can be of two types:
  a) Non specific
  b) Immunologic

VII. THE FUNDAMENTAL FEATURES OF IMMUNE RESPONSE:

1. IMMUNE SPECIFICITY:

Immune response against any antigen is two fold. First an immediate non specific response. Second is a delayed specific response.

Delayed response is due to production of specific Antibodies (Humoral Immune response) & production of sensitized calls (CMI) which kill specific antigen.

The basis of Immuno specificity is, specific configuration of Antibodies and Antigenic determinants present over antigen delineating its specificity.

I. HUMORAL IMMUNITY:

- Cells responsible are B Lymphocytes (B Cells). B Cells are produced in Bursae of fabricius equivalent bone marrow in human body. When specific Antigen is presented to B Cells, dominant clones of B Cells specific to that Antigen enlarge and differentiate into lymphoblast, plasmoblast and plasma cells which produce specific Antibodies against that specific Antigen

- Antibodies (Gamma globin proteins) are basic units of humoral immunity. There are five types of Antibodies IgG/IgA/IgM/IgD/IgE

II. CELLULAR IMMUNITY (CMI OR CELL MEDIATED IMMUNITY)

- Cellular basis of CMI is T Lymphocyte (T Cells). T Cells are present in peripheral lymphoid tissue as well as in circulating blood. T Cells consist 70-80% of all lymphocyte, are produced in Thymus and have two functions cellular immune reaction and regulation of immune response

- Cellular immune reaction Which is highly specific and acts via killer cells to cause Delayed Hypersensitivity, Resistance against tumors and Rejection of solid organ transplants

2. IMMUNOLOGIC MEMORY:

i) Primary Response:

When an antigen is exposed for the first in body, an immune response is launched after some delay (latent period) this response then reaches a maximum, plateaus and later declines.

ii) Secondary Response:

When same antigen enters the body again Latent Period is less, Immune response is more, Plateau is prolonged and decline in immunity is delayed. The basis of Secondary Response is production of memory cells.

VIII. ACTIVATION OF IMMUNE RESPONSE

- The immediate reaction to invasion by an Antigen, is largely a matter of antibodies already circulating in the blood
- In the next phase which involves specific Humoral and Cell Mediated Immunities. The macrophage plays a key role
- The Macrophage primes, processes and presents the antigen molecules to both T Cells and B Cells
- B Cells are transformed into Plasma cell which produce specific antibodies (Ig) and memory B cell which become dormant

- T cell are transformed and these transformed T Cells have two functions they differentiate into different types of T Cells & secrete lymphokines which have specific function
- T cells differentiate into Helper T Cell. Suppressor T Cells, Killer T Cell & Memory T Cell
- Thus Both B and T Cells are programmed to deal with the particular antigen
- The effectiveness of the immune reaction varies from one individual to another irrespective of the type of Antigen. This suggests a genetic influence. It may be related to the HLA complex and further investigation in this field is on
- There are systems involved in an immune reaction: Humoral Immunity. Cell mediated immunity. Phagocytic Activity and Complement fixation

ACTIVATION OF SPECIFIC IMMUNE RESPONSE

4 SYSTEMS ARE INVOLVED:

i. PHAGOCYTOSIS
ii. COMPLEMENT FIXATION
iii. HUMORAL IMMUNITY
iv. CMI

IX. EFFECTOR MECHANISMS OF IMMUNE RESPONSE

- The basic reaction is the combination of Antigen (Ag) and Antibody (Ab) to from Ag-Ab complexes which cause Immediate & Delayed reactions

- Humoral Antibodies are already present in blood & tissues, therefore rapid Ag-Ab reaction takes place which is called Immediate reaction
- Cellular Antibodies depend on Lymphocyte transformation, mobilization and multiplication. This takes time of a few days and therefore called as Delayed Reaction

IMMEDIATE REACTIONS

- There are several consequences of the basic Antigen-Antibody combination which have been extensively studied in vitro these are:

1. Precipitation: where soluble Antigen is rendered insoluble.
2. Agglutination: particulate Antigen (Bacteria & RBC) are aggregated in the same way as precipitation.
3. Anti-toxic effect: The Antigen-Antibody combination neutralizes the toxic activity of the antigen.
4. Enhancement of the natural non-specific defence mechanism occurs by two ways. Increase of Macrophage activity i.e. by Phagocytosis and by Complement Activation. (a) Phagocytosis: Antigen-Antibody complex attaches to specific receptor on macrophage via the antibody. Then there is rapid adherence of antigen to the macrophage and macrophage engulfs the antigen (cell drinking) which is called as Phagocytosis.

Phagocytosis is carried out primarily by:

1. Monocyte-Macrophages
2. PMN's (Polymorpho-Neutrophils)
3. Eosinophils

Table 5: Mediator Cells & Chemotaxis

CELL TYPE	Chemotactic Factor	Cell Product
MACRO PHAGE	MIF/LMPHOKINE	Process Antigen
PMN	Lymphokine Complement associated Bacterial Factor	Kinnin SRS-A Bask Peptides
EOSINOPHILS	Lymphokine Complement Associated Bacterial Factor	ECF-A

(b) Complement Activation: Humoral immune reaction involve activation of the complement system (a 20 enzyme cascade of which 9 components are present in blood and tissue fluids) the ultimate objective of complement system i.e. Classical pathway is most commonly activated by the Ag-Ab combination via IgG and IgM antibodies, it is rapid and efficient Alternative pathway is activated by IgA and IgE also by endotoxin produced by certain bacteria and properdin, present in blood & tissues fluids.

Table 6: Complement System

Activity	Component	Result
Anaphylactic	C_{3a}, C_{5a}	Increased vascular permeability
Chemotactic	$C_{ea}, C_{5a}, C5_{67}$	Attracts cells to are of
Phagocytic	C_{3a}	Promoter Phagocytosis
Lytic	C_1-a	Perforator cell membrane

DELAYED REACTIONS

- Unlike B Cells. T Cells have complex functions, acting by two ways firstly by direct destruction of antigen laden cells and secondly by influencing other cells of immune response by the means of lymphokines. In a sense T Cells exert and overall control of the immune response
- Antigen when exposed to T cell pool, specific T Cell clones are activated which are called as transformed T Cells
- Transformed T Cell secrete growth inhibitory factor which decreases lymphocyte formation. Mitogenic factor which increase lymphocyte formation both of these extend control of lymphocyte production according to demand. Transfer factor which sensitises unsensitized lymphocyte and makes them capable of secreting mediators. Chemotactic factor for polymorph which cause migration of polymorphs to reaction site. Leucocyte inhibitory factor which limits extent of migration and concentrates WBC at the reaction site. Chemotactic and Activation factor for macrophage which induces phagocytosis via macrophage. Migration inhibitory factor which inhibits immigration of macrophages and concentrates them at reaction site. Pro coagulant factor this acts as substitute of factor VIII and helps in forming a fibrin barrier helping to limit inflammation. Interferon which helps to prevent viral infection. Colony stimulating factor which is also produced by macrophage & PMN's which aids marrow stem cells to differentiate into granulocyte and monocytes
- Transformed T Cells differentiate into Cytotoxic T Cells (K Cells) which directly kills antigen laden cell by adding pore forming enzyme Perforins on cell membrane causing lysis of cell and by directly activating programmed cell death (PCD)
- T helper cells are those which promote B cell activity thus increasing Antibody protection

- T Suppressor Cell inhibits B Cell activity there by decreasing Antibody production
- The balance of these two cells controls Humoral immune reaction to suit condition in vivo

X. REGULATION OF IMMUNE RESPONSE

- By T Cells secreting lymphokines
- T helper Cells which facilitate immune response
- T suppressor Cell which terminate immune response.
- Types of organism which activate CMI are, slowly developing bacterial disease (e.g. tubercular bacillus). Cancer Cells, Transplant Cells, Fungus & Viruses

Figure 1: **MACROPHAGE PRIMES AND PRESENT AG TO IMMUNE SYSTEM**

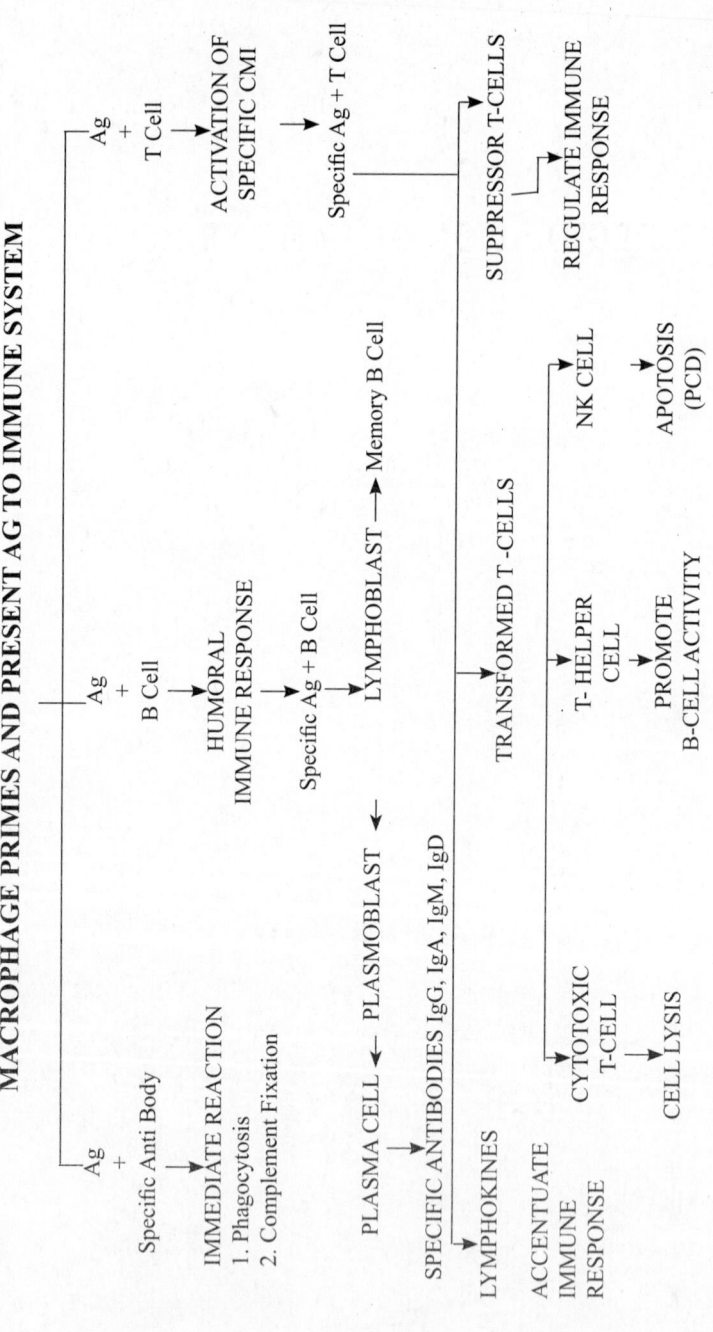

Chapter 17

Concept of Immunologic Balance

- The immunologic system maybe viewed as a system of cells & cell products whose main function is the recognition & destruction of foreign material.
- The efficacy of this removal will determine if the net result that is: Beneficial (IMMUNITY) or harmful (HYPERSENSITIVITY)
- Let us now construct a working hypothesis of interaction of the various components between:
  1. ENVIRONMENT
  2. TARGET CELLS
  3. PHAGOCYTIC; MEDIATOR; SAR-CELLS
- Following confrontation of Antigen there is a disequilibrium in the host
- Immunologic balance is then restored by an appropriate set of immunologic responses involving this multipotential system
- Total Immunogenic response of the Host can be divided as:
  1. PRIMARY (Non-Specific)

2. SECONDARY (Specific)
3. TERTIARY (Tissue injuring response)

- Primary response is inflammation or detoxification mechanisms
- If there is successful elimination of antigen at this step secondary and tertiary responses are not launched and the invading antigen is successfully eliminated
- If antigen persists then primary immune response processes this antigen and against this processed antigen secondary immune response is launched
- This secondary immune response is specific immune response
- The immediate secondary immune reaction is called immediate reaction the basis of which is Humoral immunity. This is formation of Ag-Ab complexes by Humoral antibodies present already in blood
- Ag-Ab complexes are removed by phagocytosis or they activate the complement system
- Ag-Ab complexes also activate a Delayed secondary immune response, which is called Delayed reaction the basis of which is Cell Mediated immunity or CMI. Cellular antibodies depends upon lymphocyte transformation, mobilization & multiplication this takes a few days time and hence called Delayed reaction
- By the time secondary Immune response is over invading antigens are successfully eliminated and there is no organic immune damage to the organism
- If secondary immune response fails to successfully eliminate the invading antigen then Tertiary immune response is launched in a last ditch effort to eliminate antigen but Tertiary immune response leads to immunologically mediated diseases of man
- These are five immunologically mediated diseases called as Type 1 to Type V Hypersensitivity reaction

Table 7: Concept of Immunologic Balance

Primary	Secondary		Tertiary
Inflammatory Response and Phagocytosis	Specific Immune Response		Immunologic Mediated Diseases of Man
Processed Ag	Humoral		
		IgE	Type I Disease
		Complement	Type II Disease
		IgM; IgG	Type III
		Cell Mediated Immunity	Type IV Disease
			Type V Disease

Figure 2: Schematic representation of the total immunologic capability of the host.

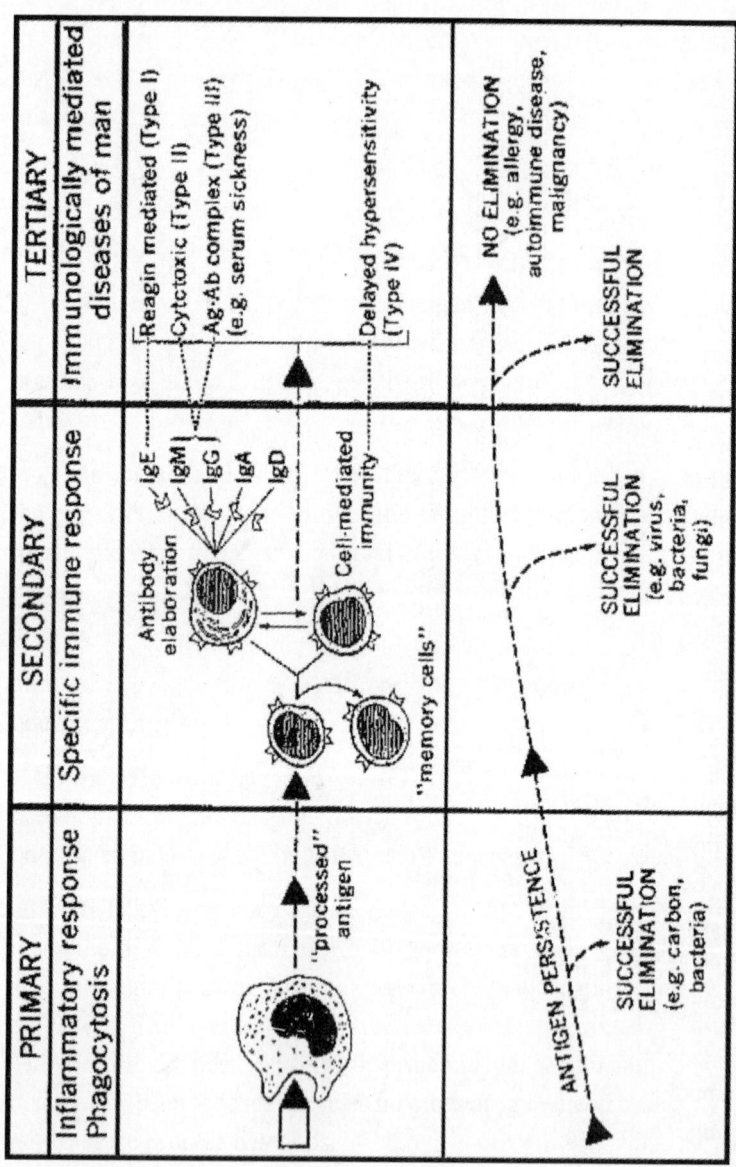

Chapter 18

Immunity & Diseases[36,33,50]

The normal function of immune system is essential for health, dysfunction of immune system leads to wide variety of diseases. Deficiency of immune cell production or defective immune cell function can lead to a spectrum of Immune Deficiency Disease, Overactivity of various components of Immune system leads to the development of allergic and Auto Immune disease. Malignant transformation in cell of immune system leads to Leukemia and Lymphoma.

The host defense system is divided into two major categories: Non immune defense system and Immune defense system. Non immune defense is not antigen specific and begins within minutes of an invasion and does not have memory for the eliciting stimulus this process is called Inflammation. Neutrophils, Eosinophils, Basophils, NK cells. Monocyte and Macrophage are mediators of this immediate response system, they also play a key role in development of subsequent immune response.

The Immune defense system consists of Humoral and Cellular Immunity the principle effector of cellular immunity is thymus derived Lymphocyte (T Cell) and of Humoral immunity is the bone marrow derived, bursae equivalent lymphocyte (B Cell). Other key effector &

regulatory cells of the immune system are Lymphocytes and Monocyte Macrophages.

MECHANISM OF IMMUNE DAMAGE

In this scenario, the classic weapons of immune system T cell, B cell and Macrophages interact with cells & soluble products which are mediators of inflammatory response.

There are four general phases of host defense. Migration of Leukocytes to sites of Antigen relocalization. Specific and non specific Recognition of foreign antigens mediated by T&B lymphocytes macrophages and Alternative complement pathway. Amplification of inflammatory response by complement components, lymphokines, kinins prostaglandins, mast cell and basophil products. Macrophage, Neutrophil, T-cell and B-cell participation in antigen Destruction with ultimate removal of Antigen particle by phagocytosis or by direct cytotoxic mechanism.

Under normal circumstances, orderly progression of host defense through these phases results in well controlled Immune and Inflammatory response that protects the host from the offending antigen. However, dysfunction of any of the host defense system can damage host tissue and produce clinically apparent disease furthermore for certain pathogen or antigens the normal immune response itself might contribute substantially to the tissue damage.

The complicated and delicately balanced immune mechanism has been developed to protect against antigens, particularly infections. When these immune reactions are upset the protective mechanism can itself be a source a disease states.

There are three main categories:

1. Hypersensitive reactions or exaggerated immune response

2. Immune deficiency conditions
3. Auto immune diseases

1. HYPERSENSITIVE REACTIONS (EXAGGERATED IMMUNE RESPONSE)

Basically these consist of an exaggerated response by an individual to an antigen, following a previous exposure. The resulting Ag-Ab reaction induces the release of large quantities of chemicals, enzymes and cell stimulators. Depending on the type of immune response concerned these hypersensitivity reactions are classified as follows:

a. Those associated with humoral antibodies which occur within 24 hours therefore called immediate hypersensitivity reactions. These are further subdivided into type I, type II, type III and type V.

b. Those associated with cell medicated immunity are called as delayed hypersensitivity reactions because they occur after 24-72 hours. These are also known as type IV hypersensitivity reaction.

This classification is to some extent artificial, Hypersensitivity may start as an immediate humoral reaction but end in a mixed state with both humoral and cell medicated activity.

TYPE I REACTION OR ANAPHYLAXIS OR ATOPY OR ALLERGY

The basic mechanism is that after first exposure to Ag there is formation of IgE which is fixed to mast cells and basophils. On subsequent exposure to the same antigen there occurs an antigen-antibody reaction on the surface of mast cell which leads to degranulation of mast cell from which there is release of mediators of inflammation and vasoactive amines which ultimately manifested as

Anaphylaxis or Allergic reaction. Clinical example of Type I reaction are Anaphylactic shock, Hay fever, Asthma.

Basic Mechanism in type I reaction is increased production of IgE. Allergic conditions are often familial and with genetic basis. Allergens are antigens which induce allergic reaction common examples are Anti-tetanus serum, penicillin, bee venom, pollen, house mite, dust, and food drugs etc.

TYPE II REACTION OR CYTOTOXIC REACTION

Antigen is on the cell surface which combines with specific antibody to produce complement activation which increases phagocytosis (opsonic effect) and increase killer cell activity, the net effect is destruction of cell over which antigen is present. Clinical examples are transfusion reactions and Hemolytic anemia.

TYPE III REACTION OR ARTHUS REACTION

This reaction is due to the consequences of specific direct Antigen-Antibody combination, particularly compliment activation and platelet aggregation. The antibodies involved are commonly IgG and IgM. Antigen-Antibody complex cause compliment activation which in turn causes release of vasoactive amines which have effect on vessel wall. The compliment activation also leads to chemotaxis of polymorph, this along with platelet aggregation leads to thrombus formation at the site of Antigen-Antibody reaction In Arthus reaction Antigen-Antibody complex do not cause hypersensitivity but they aggregate in small vessels and with complement cause tissue destruction. Clinical example being serum sickness.

TYPE IV OR CELL MEDIATED OR DELAYED HYPERSENSITIVITY

This is due to specifically sensitized T cells. Antigen release toxins which cause immediate inflammation, 24-72 hours after this there is infiltration by sensitized T cells, which either swell up to form Granuloma or they destroy the antigen, this is known as delayed reaction. The clinical examples are Tubercular granuloma, rashes of viral infection, contact dermatitis, rejection of graft.

TYPE V OR STIMULATORY TYPE

This is a modification of Type II reaction in which specific antibody combines with Ag on the cell surface but this complex (Ag-Ab) does not activate complement but mimics the action of Physiological agent which would normally turn on the activity of the cell. Clinical example is Grave's disease (Exophthalmic goitre).

2. IMMUNE DEFICIENCY STATES

Four systems are involved in an immune reactions: Humoral Antibody System, CMI, Phagocytic Defense & Complement Fixation. Failure in one of these alters the immune response. The deficiencies may be of primary nature, commonly genetic in nature or secondary to some other diseases or circumstances. Clinically all immune deficiencies are characterized by chronic or recurring infections caused by ordinary commensals.

Humoral Deficiency:

This may be result of lack of B lymphocyte, inability of B cells to secrete immunoglobulins or due to increased activity of suppressor mechanism. Examples of humoral deficiency are X linked hypogammaglobulinemia and IgA deficiency.

CMI Deficiency:

Two Type seen, congenital (Di George's Syndrome) and Acquired (AIDS)

Combined B & T Cell Deficiency:

Which is genetic and rare

Phagocytic Deficiency:

Which is of two Type:

Primary, due to defect in phagocytic enzymes, resulting in inability to kill and digest bacteria this is called as Chronic Granulomatous disease.

Another type of primary phagocytic deficiency may be due to defective response of Phagocytes to chemotactic stimuli, Called as Lazy leucocyte syndrome.

Secondary Phagocytic deficiency is due to abnormal chemotactic factors, immunosuppressive drug therapy, autoimmunity against Phagocyte.

Compliment Deficiency:

Although rare if present it is frequently a cause of an Autoimmune reaction.

3. AUTO IMMUNE DISEASES

Auto immune diseases result from or are associated with an immune response against the individuals own cells, or in some cases cell products. It involves changes in Humoral, CMI and in Tolerance. The etiology of Auto immune diseases is not established but clues to their genesis are available.

The basic cause of Auto immune diseases seems to be inborn instability of immune tolerance and changes is immune mechanism there by involve four factors which are constantly active. Altered cell antigens cause B cell stimulation, T helper stimulation, T killer cell activation which leads to proliferation of B cell, increased antibody production, Antigen-Antibody complex formation and complement fixation but there is a lack of T suppressor cell activity thereby causing uncontrolled tissue destruction.

The absence of T cell suppressor controls remains unexplained & seems to be the key to Autoimmune pathogenesis examples of Autoimmune diseases are Hashimotos disease, Pernicious anemia, hemolytic anemia, NIDDM, Vitiligo etc.

Chapter 19

Immunity and Homoeopathy[13,19,22,24,26,27,30,42,44,47,50]

PATTERSON ON IMMUNITY AND HOMOEOPATHY

I would like you to note that it was only after a period of experience in the practice of Homoeopathy – that is the treatment of disease according to the Law of Similars – that is was forced to give consideration to the Hahnemannian Doctrine of the Psoric Miasm.

It is possible to practice homoeopathy without any knowledge of the Hahnemannian doctrine. I shall be commenting on this later in this paper. Meantime let me recall for you a common experience in the homoeopathic treatment of acute disease in children.

A child is admitted to hospital, acutely and dangerously ill, with Broncho-pneumonia. From the symptom complex-not from the name of the disease-a remedy is selected, and homoeopathic treatment is given, for this case of Broncho-pneumonia. Within a short period of hours there is evidence of improvement in the child's condition, and finally the symptoms of Broncho-pneumonia disappear-the child is cured.

That, however, is not the happy ending of the story, for in 14 days time, when the parents visit the "cured" child they are horrified to find it covered in an unsightly skin eruption, and naturally demand an explanation. At the bedside, in the presence of the junior medical or nursing staff, one may ease one's conscience by demonstrating the case as an excellent example of the manifestation of the basic miasm of Psora, but in the waiting room, before the parents, it requires considerable courage to expound the doctrine of Hahnemann and convince them, that because of this eruptive condition, their child is now in a much healthier condition than when admitted.

The sequel, not infrequently, is the removal of the child by the indignant parents, and not only so, but the parents or the child in the next cot demand that their child be removed from contact with a child suffering from a dirty skin disease. All this, please note, is the result of the homoeopathic treatment of acute illness and the manifestation of the underlying Psoric Miasm of Hahnemann.

Before further discussion I must confess that I accept as my standard reference the English translation by Charles. J. Hempel published in 4 volumes in New York, 1845, "The Chronic Diseases- their Nature and Homoeopathic Treatment."This, I think, is the only English translation available and I was much encouraged by Hempel's introductory remarks.

He says "Hahnemann's phraseology is so involved and bears so little resemblance to the usual mode of constructing periods, either in German or any other language, that it is utterly impossible to furnish a bare translation of Hahnemann's writings." He then adds this sentence, "I have not translated words but ideas." That, in my opinion, is the only method of translating Hahnemann's writings and so getting to know the fundamental ideas upon which he formulated his doctrines.

Throughout the homoeopathic literature, you will find, here and there, extracts from the context of "Chronic Diseases" by authors who attempt to make literal translation, each making a different sense and, in the end, confusing the student who attempts to find the true basis of the Hahnemannian doctrine.

I shall be making reference to some of these extracts and commenting on how they digress from the basic ideas of Hahnemann. My interpretation of Hahnemann's ideas must therefore depend upon the English translation by Charles. J. Hempel, M.D., and I shall quote his text as the basis of my comments.

I want to make this point quite clear-to state my source of information-as there has been so much controversy as to what Hahnemann did or did not say regarding the Miasm.

This controversy began almost as soon as the published "The Chronic Diseases" It would seem that this controversy still goes on. In 1837 it is recorded that Central Congress of homoeopaths held at Frankfort-am-Main, a resolution was passed condemning the Hahnemannian Doctrine, and in the Pacific Coast Homoeopathic Bulletin of January, 1953 you will find an article entitled "Discounting Hahnemann's theory of Miasms's."

This later paper by Harvey Farrington is in answer to a previous one by a Dr. Renner in which he concluded that "we do not find anything added since Hahnemann's time and that his theory of miasms is altogether without foundation in fact." It will be evident from the context of this paper that I do not agree with that conclusion, and I shall be giving you factual evidence, which not only adds to, but supports, the doctrine of Hahnemann.

I should like you to note that it was the result of his observations in the practice of Homoeopathy, that led him to a new conception as to the nature of disease and the publication of the Organon in 1810. This publication I suggest might be called the "Beginners' Handbook" to the study of the Doctrine of Hahnemann.

May I briefly summarize the main points in the teaching of Hahnemann as expressed in the Organon.

First, and I think of greatest importance, is his conception the existence of a "vital force" capable of maintaining life itself, of maintaining normal function and sensation; a force capable of adjusting itself to internal or external influences:-this he called "DYNAMIS."

Should anything disturb this balance, the action of the Dynamis would produce abnormal functioning and abnormal sensation, a symptom complex which should be interpreted as the evidence of disease, and not as the prime disease.

I find that it is difficult for the modern medical student to grasp the significance of this conception of the nature of disease, so may I break this sequence to give an example. The treatment would follow one's conception as to the nature of the disease present, and as we are considering skin diseases let us take the case of a skin eruption. Upon the diagnosis will depend the rationale of treatment. If the skin eruption is declared to be an Exfoliative Dermatitis-based on the pathological evidence-the treatment must be local treatment of the skin. If, however, the diagnosis is that the eruption is the evidence of an internal condition-a manifestation of the psoric miasm-then treatment must be directed to the prime cause-the miasm.

Hahnemann, from his experience of Homoeopathy, declared that Nature had no nomenclature for disease; that it was unscientific to treat disease according to the nomenclature based on pathology.

In logical sequence, therefore, we find that "the sole guide to direct us in the choice of a remedy must be the sum total of all the symptoms and conditions in each individual case of disease." (§ 18-Organon.)

In his clinical observations Hahnemann found it necessary to divide diseases into (1) Acute and (2) Chronic –which he defines for us (§ 72-Organon).

ACUTE Disease: is characterized by "rapid morbid processes which have a tendency to finish their course more or less quickly.

CHRONIC Disease: is characterized by imperceptible beginnings, gradual onset, so that the vital force, whose office is to preserve the health, offers imperfect resistance and becomes ever more and more abnormally deranged.

CHRONIC Disease: are caused by dynamic infection with a chronic miasm.

I have paraphrased this paragraph from the text of the 6th Edition of the Organon because I think it of the greatest importance and I have underlined in my script these words "vital force whose office is to preserve the health" and in the last sentence "caused by dynamic infection with a chronic miasm."

Let's leave Hahnemann and Homoeopathy for the moment and consider the course of an acute disease as exemplified in a case of measles. We must presume that at some particular point in time, the virus infection entered the child's body, and in 10 days time there developed the typical symptoms, followed by the appearance of a characteristic skin eruption (rash) on the 14th day.

That the symptoms can be acute and even endanger a child's life will be agreed by all who have experience of this disease, but the remarkable point in the course of the majority of the cases, is the rapid easing of the acute symptoms and the comparative quick recovery immediately after the appearance of the rash.

Experimental evidence into the production of immunity, shows that the tissues are not dormant in the incubation period, but highly active. There are three factors concerned in the production of immunity and the cure of the acute exanthematous disease.

1. The body cells must produce, fix, then eliminate the virus to complete the cure.
2. All body cells possess the ability to produce anti-toxin but there is a considerable difference in the degree of production.

The skin possesses this capability to the highest degree and the blood plasma to the least degree.

3. While all cells have the potential to produce anti-toxin, not all have the power to fix the anti-toxin, that is to make a physico-chemical union, and finally by a process of proteolysis destroy the virus (Tissue Immunity-Kaha.)

Applying this experimental evidence to the actual case of measles, we can reason this. The virus enters the body, affecting local cells, which have the power to produce to a higher or lower degree anti-toxin, but lacking the power to fix the toxin, it can only at best put up a local defense, the living virus goes on producing its toxin, even during the incubation period, and it is only when the blood plasma has been sufficiently saturated that the toxin reaches the skin with its high degree of anti-toxin production and power to make a physico-chemical union and finally proteolyse the virus of measles.

The skin eruption is the result of the physico-chemical disturbance taking place in the skin cells which have the power to fix and destroy the toxin-the whole phenomenon is a measure of the defensive power mechanism of the body, and evidence of an inherent vital force, whose function it is to maintain a state of health.

Meantime we have noted that, in acute exanthematous disease-there is a vital force which comes into action and, as a defensive measure, the skin has to play an important role. As a result of this skin disturbance, the disease is eliminated and health restored in a comparatively short period of time. Also, let us keep in mind, that there is a latent period from the time infection until the evidence of the full defensive action on the skin the incubation period.

It is clear from his writings, that Hahnemann did foresee the contagions of certain diseases, Small-pox and Malaria, and had in mind infection of the body by "parasitic living animalcule" but the terms of his day are capable of different interpretation today as a result of the work of Pasteur and his disciples. Today the word "parasitic" simply implies a living plant or animal living in the tissues of another living plant or animal-it is not necessarily associated with disease, it may be symbiotic: for example, the B. Coli of the intestinal canal, may even be beneficial to host.

If you are looking for modern scientific data to support the practice of Homoeopath, and the soundness of the Hahnemannian teachings, I suggest that you read up any modern text book on the subject of "Immunity."

Now we must return to the Organon and Hahnemann's writings on Chronic Disease, and in Para. 78 we find clearly stated that "the true natural chronic disease are those that arise from a chronic miasm."

In the footnote 76, he gives an example of the action of this chronic miasm, in which he assumes that the miasm is present at birth, but this may not be evident during "the flourishing years of youth" but, later, the first symptoms appear and develop in speed and severity, in proportion to the external stress or worry to which the vital principle is exposed. In this you will note that Hahnemann recognizes two factors (1) internal (Heredity) and (2) external (Environment).

In my interpretation of the Hahnemannian idea, I reserve the term "Dynamis" to indicate in general terms the vital force operating from the moment of birth and continuing under the most favourable circumstances to maintain normal function – that is to maintain a state of health.

MIASM can be defined as a form of DERANGED DYNAMIS– that vital force working under adverse circumstances, and failing to maintain normal function, and thus producing the symptom-complex we call DIS-ease.

In the original use of the word, miasm was the vapour or mist which the earlier physicians associated with the incidence of Malaria– they considered this to be the cause of the disease.

Now of course we know that the "miasm" was but the breeding ground for the mosquito and its infective malaria germ, but the word was adapted by Hahnemann to indicate, not any external factor, but one which is inherent in the living cell, a deranged vital force.

It is this inherent deranged vital force which produces the disease, and so it becomes possible for the physician, by his "taking of the Case" to get some indication as to the degree of the deranged dynamis – to recognize the type of MIASM.

It is appropriate that we consider the miasm which Hahnemann called Psora which we find described in § 80 (Organon).

The paragraph is again a very complicated one and difficult to follow in the original text, but I shall try to translate truly the idea of Hahnemann. There are two points of fundamental importance in this paragraph in the identification of Psoric Diseases.

1. A peculiar skin eruption characterized by intolerable itching.
2. This skin eruption appears AFTER THE COMPLETION OF THE INTERNAL INFECTION OF THE WHOLE ORGANISM. Once again we find a footnote 77 in which, from his clinical experience over a period of 12 years, he states that he was not able to treat the chronic diseases as isolated individual maladies, even by the most careful application of the Law of Similars. Wherein lay the cause of this failure to get permanent results in chronic disease. That could be investigated under three heads.

   i. Failure in the Law of Similars as applied to chronic disease-that it was nor a universal law of therapeutics.

   ii. Failure because of limitation in the number of remedies available or lack of knowledge of their action.

   iii. Failure to obtain the totality of the symptoms of the disease.

Under (i) failure of the Law of Similars, it was evident that on occasion the law did work well, at other times indifferently or not at all. It could not be this factor which caused failure.

The work of Hahnemann represented by the 6 volumes of his Materia Medica is sufficient evidence that he fully investigated this factor, but did not find the solution to his immediate problem-the treatment of chronic disease.

The answer he found under the third heading (Pg 87)-failure to obtain the totality of the symptoms. Hahnemann realised that the chronic disease are but phases of a chronic miasm. To apply successfully the law of Similars one must find a remedy to cover not only the immediate symptoms of the acute phase but also "all the ailments and symptoms inherent in the unknown primitive malady." (Chronic Disease, Vol. 1)

In my earlier experience in the practice of Homoeopathy, based entirely upon the Law of Similars, I found as Hahnemann did, that I was unable to get the result which one would expect to get in the more chronic type of disease, from the application of what one believed to be a universal and a scientific form of therapeutics.

My observations on the bowel flora, and the clinical success which seemed to follow the use of the bowel nosodes, led me to accept the more readily the doctrine of Hahnemann expressed in the words I have already quoted from Organon: "Chronic disease are caused by dynamic infection with a chronic miasm."

In this quotation, the use of the phrase "dynamic infection" has led many to interpret the meaning as it would apply today-that infection implies invasion of the body by a living germ or virus, but it is clear from the example given in his introduction of the Organon, the effect of psychological shock as coming under the phrase "dynamic infection." He speaks of "an irritating word bringing on a dangerous bilious fever."

CHRONIC DISEASES are thus to be considered as due to an inherited MIASM a deranged dynamis – which manifests its action during the lifetime of the individual by a variety of symptom complexes.

Following up the example of Hahnemann, I examined all the possible causes of failure and arrived at the conclusion that it was not the Law of Similars which has failed me, but my own failure to ascertain the totality of the symptoms.

I recalled the second of the fundamental points of the Organon, that "this skin eruption appears AFTER THE COMPLETION OF THE INTERNAL INFECTION OF THE WHOLE ORGANISM"- note these words, "after the completion of the internal infection." That would imply that the skin eruption was the sequel, the terminal phase of an internal infection, and again my mind turned to the analogy of the acute exanthemata, to the various phases seen, as for example, in case of measles.

After a definite dynamic infection with a living virus, there was a period, the incubation period, during which there was no evidence of disease, but in 10 days time the first symptoms, the prodromal symptoms of Measles were manifested, and after a further period-4 days the typical measles rash appeared. No one would suggest that the typical rash represented the totality of the symptom complex of the disease-Measles, and so it should be in the taking of the case in the case in the psoric skin eruption –the skin characteristics do not constitute the totality of the symptoms of the disease. There is a prodromal period with first evidence of abnormal function and sensation, and it is these symptoms which give the more accurate picture of the disease. It is a fact that the more advanced the disease-the presence of marked pathological change-the less evident are the initial characteristic symptoms by which the homoeopath physician identifies the disease and chooses the most similar remedy.

I trust that you may have followed my reasoning and will accept my conclusion, that in the homoeopathic treatment of skin disease, the physician must take the full clinical history of the case, laying the greater importance on the symptoms which preceded the eruption on the skin as a guide to the most similar remedy.

I attribute my earlier failures in the treatment of skin diseases to the fact that I concentrated on the finding of a remedy which had the greatest similarity to the characteristics of the skin eruption. There are so many psoric remedies which have common symptoms in their terminal action on the skin, that I suggest that in taking the case of a skin eruption, you give the apparently outstanding skin characteristics second place and give first rank to the finer symptoms in the clinical history which may have preceded the skin eruption by a considerable time period.

In the example of the measles case, there is a definite time period of incubation, from infection to the appearance of the rash, but in the psoric skin eruptions this time period varies so considerably for each individual, and if we accept the Hahnemannian conception, the dynamic infection or affection of the vital force-the Dynamis-dates from birth. Chronic diseases owe their origin to an inherent chronic miasm.

In the taking of a case of psoric skin eruption one must presume that the prodromal period dates from birth and note the various disturbances which may have taken place from then up to the date of the eruption.

In such a clinical history, there may be acute illnesses, acute in the sense that they are severe and may endanger life, but in the Hahnemannian conception they are but acute phases of the underlying chronic miasm.

It is these phases in the clinical history which may give you the clue to the basic miasm, and lead to the choice of the most similar remedy in the treatment of the skin eruption.

The first point to note is, that in Psora, the skin eruption must be considered to be "chronic," and in this category it requires a special from of treatment. When you are next called upon to treat an acute eczema, please keep this point in mind, it is "chronic"in the Hahnemannian sense.

I think you will agree that, in such a case, it is of the utmost importance to do everything possible to lessen the intolerable itching-provided that such measures do not interfere with the treatment of the basic miasm.

I warned you earlier not to pay too much attention to the choice of the most similar remedy to the skin eruption, in the treatment of the basic miasm-that the skin remedy would not bring about the cure even of the skin eruption. The outbreak on the skin, we have noted, is the result of the defensive action of the body, the fixing of the toxin by the skin cells, by a physico-chemical combination, hence the pathological change.

According to rule, this change, this end result, requires the giving of a low potency-6c. or lower, and frequent repetition, and in practice I have found that the choice of the most suitable remedy for the skin symptom, although it does not clear the eruption, has power to lessen the itching, because it is homoeopathic to skin lesion.

At the same time, one must treat the basic, and the choice of the remedy must be taken from the acute phases, the earlier symptoms, and potency level would be from the 30 CH. upwards, going higher and higher as necessary and repeating at intervals as indicated by the clinical changes observed.

In this way I think you will find greater clinical success in the treatment of skin diseases, and also in other forms of chronic disease.

I cannot close this paper without a word about the significance of the skin eruption in relation to Hahnemann's Doctrine of Psora.

Modern immunology accepts the phenomenon of skin eruption as indicative of the defensive mechanism of the body, and the extent of skin eruption reflects the degree of immunity than those without.

It is a well observed fact that the diseases with marked skin eruption develop a greater immunity than those without.

Compare the immunity following Scarlet Fever, Measles, etc., with the increased susceptibility which seems to follow an attack of the virus disease of influenza.

Even in acute disease it is a clinical fact that, if the skin does not erupt sufficiently to fix and totally destroy the toxin, and internal disease may remain, e.g., the Nephritis which may be left behind in Scarlet Fever.

In Chronic Disease, according to the Hahnemannian conception, the inherent vital force is unable of its own accord to set in motion the specialized defensive mechanism possessed by the skin cells.

It is clear that he did realize that the skin eruption did play an important role in the cure of chronic disease, and that he regarded the appearance of a skin eruption after the giving of a remedy as of good omen, a sign of vital reaction.

I rather expect that in the discussion which is to follow, I may be questioned regarding my views on the Psora-Scabies controversy, which I hear still in some homoeopathic circles.

I can find no definite evidence that Hahnemann did specifically relate Psora to Scabies-the Itch, but that he did define Psora as characterized by a peculiar skin eruption with an intolerable itch. I think that the controversy was started by his disciples who mis-translated "an itchy skin eruption" into "the itchy skin eruption" – to the prevalent skin disease of the time-Scabies.

In any case, I think it is beside the point to argue on that, when it is so evident that he was the first physician to realize the role of the skin in the defense of the body, in the production of immunity to dynamic infection. The Hahnemannian Doctrine of Psora is based on clinical observations and scientific fact as evidenced by the present day experiments in immunology.

NIGAM ON IMMUNITY AND HOMOEOPATHY[25,50]

A. HAHNEMANN'S CONCEPT OF VITAL FORCE

- Vital force is conceptual controlling principle of life §
- *In the healthy human state, the spirit-like like force (autocracy) that enlivens the material organism as dynamis, governs without restriction and keeps all parts of the organism in admirable, harmonious, vital operation, as regards both feelings and functions, so that our indwelling, rational spirit can freely avail itself of this living, healthy instrument for the higher purposes of our existence. § 9*
- In fact Hahnemann gave another name to this conceptual controlling principle of life in (Fig. 4) Autocracy. For better understanding what Hahnemann means lets understand what we mean be democracy: (Fig. 3). It is a concept, which governs our Indian nation. It has four main pillars (1) The parliament (2) The Judiciary (3) The law enforcement agencies (4) Press.

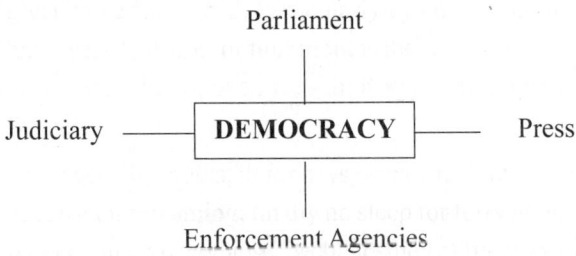

Figure 3: Attributes of Democracy

- Similarly the Autocracy (Fig. 4) has four main attributes (1) The formative forces (2) The destructive forces (3) Immunity (4) The balancing forces
- So you can't see democracy but see its effects on our nation and see it functioning through its attributes or symbols similarly

Autocracy cannot be seen (the vital principle; vital force; dynamis; wesen) but its functioning in health and deviation from health as morbid signs and symptoms which is called disease is seen, felt and perceived.

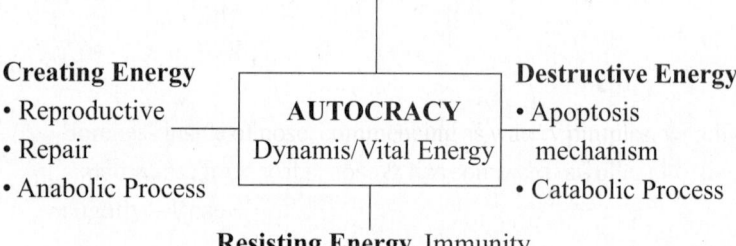

Figure 4: Attributes of Vital Force (Autocracy)

- Now we come to understand what Hahnemann means when he says the Vital force or Autocracy is the conceptual controlling principle of life. To sum vital force in a definition: "Vital force/ Dynamis/Wesen is not an organised entity or a thing or an object but is purely non material invisible inherent conceptual controlling inner force or energy that controls the molecular, chemical and mechanical processes and uses these processes for maintenance of sensation, function and for self preservation."

B. HAHNEMANN'S CONCEPT OF DISEASE

- Hahnemann classified diseases therapeutically as

    a. Indisposition (§ 150)

    b. Dynamic disease (§ 159 / § 186)

    c. Surgical disease (§ 13)

- He further subdivided Dynamic diseases into three

    a. Acute (§ 72)

b. Intermittent (§ 231)

c. Chronic disease (§ 72)

- He further subdivided chronic diseases into three

  a. Chronic diseases due to medicine (§ 74)

  b. False chronic disease (§ 77)

  c. True chronic disease or chronic miasmatic disease (§ 78)

- Diseases are nothing other than alteration of conditions in healthy people which express themselves through diseased signs i.e. Hahnemann describes diseases as dynamic mistunement of vital force. (§ 19) *"When I call disease a derangement of man's state of health, I am far from wishing thereby to give a hyper physical explanation of the internal nature of disease generally, or of any case of disease in particular. It is only intended by this expression to intimate, what it can be proved disease are not and cannot be, that they are not mechanical or chemical alterations of the material substance of the body and are not dependent on a material morbific substance, but that they are merely spirit like dynamic derangements of the life" (footnote § 31)"*.

- As fundamental cause of true chronic diseases he names three basis miasm: Internal Psora, Internal Syphilis and Internal Sycosis (§ 204)

C. PSORIC THEORY OF DISEASE

- Psora is the real fundamental cause and producer of all other numerous, I may say innumerable, forms of disease, which figures in systematic works on pathology as peculiar, independent disease (§ 80)

- Hahnemann's hypothesis was that chronic disease are chronic because some unknown devitalizing principal subverts life forces in such a way that the dynamic mistunement of health cannot be corrected. He called these unknown devitalizing principles to be chronic miasma

- The true chronic diseases according to Hahnemann were chronic miasmatic diseases. Hahnemann classified chronic miasmatic disease as two; the venereal & the non-venereal (§ 79, 80)

- The two venereal chronic miasmatic diseases were called Sycosis (the fig wart disease; typified by excrescences) & Syphilis (the chancre disease; typified by ulcer)

- To non-venereal chronic miasmatic disease he gave the name psora or the itch disease typified by pruritus

- Then Hahnemann states that the fundamental cause of all disease (including Sycosis & Syphilis) is Psora. Actually here is Hahnemann propagating his theory of causation of chronic miasmatic diseases, which Allen refers to the psoric theory of disease

- Psora is a potential that bonds itself with the life force (our inbuilt potential), that vital energy that not only animates the whole organism but sustains and controls all cell life and every physiological expression of life

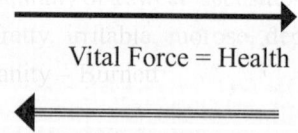

Vital Force = Health

Psoric Vital Force/Perverted Vital Force = Disease

Figure 5: Vectoral Representation of Psora & Vital Force

- By now we have also gathered that Hahnemann established psora as the cause of all illness (foundation of all sickness) so we can safely assume that psora is nothing but altered vital force, hence we can name mistuned vital force as psoric vital force

- Under the influence of perverted life action psora' life force is no longer a true dynamis but it is in bond with another dynamis, psora which knows no law and has no life giving qualities in it in fact all the dealings of psora are destructive.

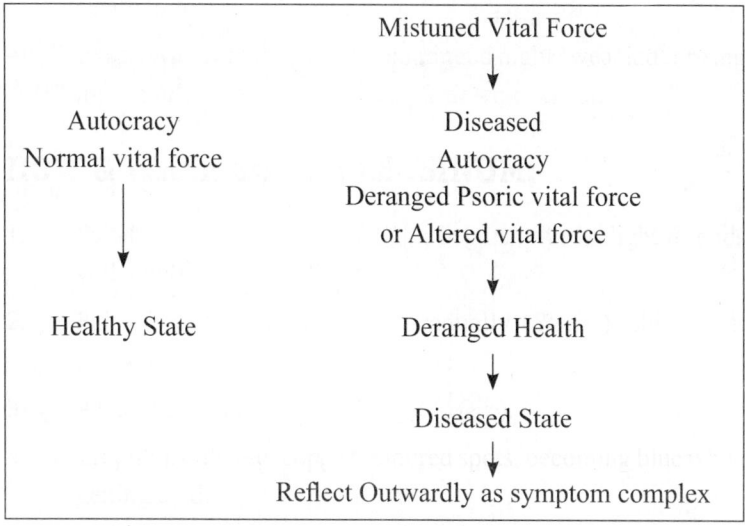

Figure 6: Comparison of Normal & Altered Vital Force

- The true internal nature of disease is thus made manifest in the study of the psoric theory of disease. Pathology can do nothing more for us today than it did in Hahnemann's time, for the simple reason that pathology is not at the bottom of that invisible process by which morbid changes and alterations take place in the organism
- It is the same with miasmatic potential; it is an invisible and unseen thing, yet we see the effects of its presence in the organism long before any changes of tissue take place
- We see it first as a rule, first manifest in the mental sphere, then in the physiological or functional, then, finally, in the pathological, the pathological, of course, coming last

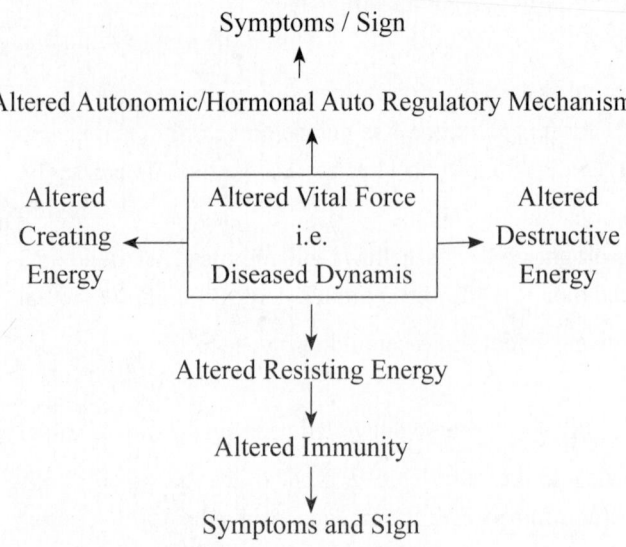

Figure 7: Attributes of Altered Vital Force

D. MIASMA AS BASIC REACTIONAL MODES OF HUMAN SYSTEM

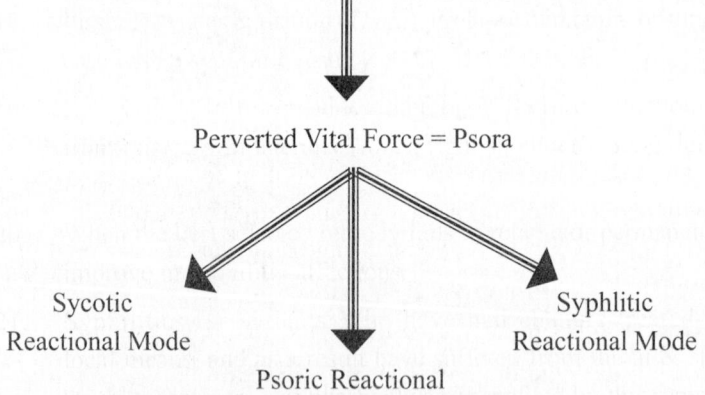

Figure 8: Three Basic Reactional Modes

- All masters quoted in section II have described in detail the effect of miasma at different level. I would like to tie together every thing under three basic reaction modes as Psora, Sycosis and Syphilis reactional mode:

  i. Psora is oscillatory or unstable relational mode

  ii. Sycosis is proliferative reactional mode

  iii. Syphilis is destructive reactional mode

  iv. Tubercular is granulomatous reactional mode

  v. Cancer is uncontrolled proliferative and destructive reactional mode

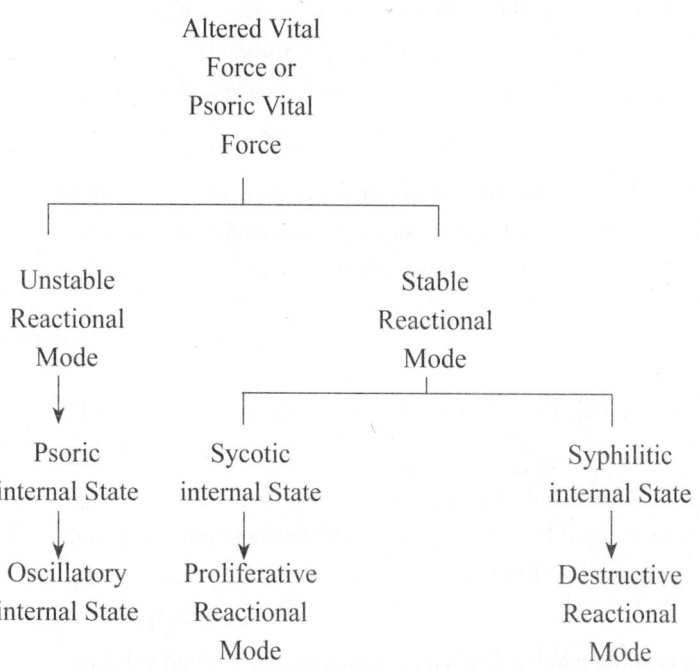

Figure 9: Three Basic Reactional Modes of Mistuned or Diseased Vital Force

- We see the landmarks of one of these chronic miasms stamped upon the organism. We see it in every feature and every physiological process; in the shape and contour of the body; upon the visual expression; we see it on the skin; by the response in the very inner being, the mental, the moral, even the spiritual, give us responses of the presence and influence of miasm
- As we become more familiar with these subversive forces in their action upon the life force, or as we see their character expressed upon the normal vitality and function of the organism, how much more easy is it for us to follow their tracings or prophesy their probable development in any given case
- If we become acquainted with the character of psora, whether expending its force upon the organism, simply, alone or in combination with some other miasm, we are more able to give a prognosis as to the probable outcome in a given case of disease; for the character and or combination of miasm gives us the character of disease or disease formula
- As we study these miasm, we see they express themselves in their degrees of action (primary, secondary and tertiary); and in their nature (acute, chronic and latent)
- We see disease to be expression of three basic potential (patho-physiological trends). He who has become acquainted with the higher homoeopathics of Hahnemann, which comprises not only of disease potentials, but the drug action, can apply the law of similia at a deeper level

E. IMMUNITY AND HOMOEOPATHY

- Since Hahnemann's time pathophysiology has moved on and now one thing is clear that in the genesis of disease, immunity is the common denominator

- It is clear now that chronic diseases as well as acute diseases are caused by disordered immunity. Even the mental diseases ruin health via immunity. This has been established by psycho-neuro-immunology
- We can explore miasma theory on the basis of immunity
    i) Altered immunity ⟶ Hypersensitivity reaction ⟶ Immuno damage ⟶ Chronic disease
    ii) Immunodeficiency state ⟶ External pathogens cause direct cellular damage ⟶ Chronic disease
- Please take note that Psoric reactional mode is an oscillatory reactional mode because it oscillates between Exaggerated immuno response (Hypersensitivity) and immuno-deficiency states
    iii) By this logic Hypersensitivity reactions are fundamentally Psoric reactional mode (Psora is the fundamental cause of all diseases-Hahnemann)

F. HYPERSENSITIVITY IMMUNO DAMAGE AND MIASMA

- Immuno damage caused by hypersensitivity leads to a spectrum of disorders there are five types of basic hypersensitivity reaction discussed in section III. The author draws similarity of five miasmas to five basic hypersensitivity reaction in the table below:

Type I	IgE Mediated Hypersensitivity	Anaphylaxis	Psoric [Itch]
Type II	Complement Mediated Hypersensitivity	Cytotoxic Reaction	Syphilitic [Cell destruction]
Type III	Igm, IgG Mediated Hypersensitivity	Arthus Reaction	Sycotic [Thrombus Formation]

Type IV	T-Cell Mediated Hypersensitivity	CMI Delayed Hypersensitivity	Tubercular [Granuloma Formation]
Type V	Ag-Ab Mediated Hypersensitivity	Stimulatory Type	Cancer [Stimulate]

Figure 10: Hypersensitivity & Miasma

G. MIASMA AS REAL CAUSE OF IMMUNOLOGIC MEDIATED DISEASES (See Figure 2: Pg No.72)

Primary	Secondary		Tertiary
Inflammatory Response and Phagocytosis	Specific Immune Response		Immunologic Mediated Diseases of Man
Processed Ag	Humoral		
		IgE	Type I Psoric Disease
		Complement	Type II Syphilitic/Leutic Disease
		IgM; IgG	Type III Sycotic Disease
		Cell Mediated Immunity	Type IV Granulomatous Disease
			Type V Cancer Disease

Figure 11: Miasma as causes of Immune Diseases

SECTION IV: POTENTIAL STUDY OF MIASMA

Chapter 20
Before Understanding the Potential Aspect of Miasma

Chapter 21
Proposed Psoric Theory of Disease

Chapter 22
Bond of Psora with Life Forces

Chapter 23
The Potential Study of Miasmatics

Chapter 24
Degree of Activity of Miasm

Chapter 25
The Miasmatic Potential

Chapter 26
Inhibitory Points

Chapter 27
The Nature of Miasm: Latent & Chronic

Chapter 20

Before Understanding Potential Aspect of Miasm[2]

In order to understand miasm, we must understand some of those fundamental principles governing homoeopathy

1. The dynamic origin of disease
2. The dynamization of drugs
3. The application of similia

Remember it was application of similia that led Hahnemann to see the miasmatic cause of disease.

He saw it was a contest between the dynamics of the drug and the dynamics of life, a battle waged by dynamized, subversive influence upon the living organism, because it resided ever in the organism and was in bond with the life.

This thought led him to look for that dynamic subversive influence which eventually precipitated as the psoric theory of disease and discovery of miasm

It is our duty to understand the genesis of human being (human order) and to observe patients. It is also our duty to understand the genesis and morphology of disease. We have consistently maintained that an acute or chronic disease in always prepared and is of always proceeded by a preliminary state (prodrome) whose origin must be sought, not in the apparent effect of microbial infection but rather in the transformation of the individual himself whose normal rhythm is gradually disturbed by various condition depending on environmental, social or professional influences, general mode of living, diet and lastly on heredity. Heredity has a profound influence on the organism and its characteristics are transmitted from generation to generation. So that the hereditary conditions under our observation should never be lost sight of. It is clear, therefore, that in the matter of treatment all these elements must be taken into account.

Chapter 21

Proposed Psoric Theory of Disease[2]

Hahnemann said that Psora was the parent or the basic element of all that is known as disease.

Hahnemann further noticed that the use of crude drugs not only produced dangerous medicinal effects, but they greatly embarrassed the life forces, complicated the diseased processes and undermined the whole organism in all directions. Especially was this true when there was present a marked Psoric or Miasmatic state, which proved to him that some ONE specific cause lay at the bottom of al chronic as well as acute, expressions of disease and this UNKNOWN, DEVITALIZING PRINCIPLE HE NAMED PSORA.

This was Hahnemann's theory while medical science accepted another theory at that time; Virchow's cellular pathology theory. Virchow's cell, the unit of life was vivified, by chemical processes or by chemical changes. At that very time Koch formulated germ theory of disease.

Hahnemann had gone all through this, had weighted & measured it, analyzed it from every standpoint, but found it wanting. He not only understood fully the unscientific workings of all the systems of medicine of his day, but he went further; he was able to prophecy the outcome and the progress & path of these systems.

For Hahnemann and Homoeopathy the guiding fundamental principles are-the dynamic origin of disease, the dynamization of drug & the application of similia.

He saw it was a contest between the dynamics of the drug and the dynamics of life, a battle waged by dynamized, subversive influence upon the living organism. Which is an unceasing thing, because it resided ever in the organism and was in bond with the life.

At times the life forces apparently free themselves from that influence, it invariably returned, often changed in expression of symptoms, but invariably it was the same old Psora, though in a new garment or new disguise.

Hahnemann's hypothesis was that chronic disease are chronic because some unknown devitalizing principle subverts life forces in such a way that the dynamic mistunement of health cannot be corrected. He called these unknown devitalizing principles to be chronic miasma.

The true chronic diseases according to Hahnemann were chronic miasmatic diseases. Hahnemann classified chronic miasmatic disease as two; the venereal & the non- venereal.

The two venereal chronic miasmatic diseases were called Sycosis (the fig wart disease; typified by excrescences) & Syphilis (the chancre disease; typified by ulcer). To non-venereal chronic miasmatic disease he gave the name psora or the itch disease typified by pruritus.

Then Hahnemann states that the fundamental cause of all disease (including Sycosis & Syphilis) is Psora. Actually here is Hahnemann propagating his theory of causation of chronic miasmatic diseases, which Allen refers to the psoric theory of disease.

Kent emphasizes psora is beginning of all physical sickness. Psora is the underlying cause, and it is this primitive or primary disorder of the human race. It is the disordered state of the internal economy of the human race. The state expresses itself in the form of various chronic manifestations, the so called chronic diseases.

Had psora never been established as a miasm upon the human race, the other chronic diseases (sycosis, syphilis, tuberculosis, cancer) would have been impossible, and susceptibility to acute diseases would also have been impossible. All the disease of mankind are built upon psora. Hence the foundation of all sickness.

In subsequent chapters we would understand the relevance of this theory. It is sufficient to say at this point of time that to the follower of Hahnemann the word psora conveys a most important meaning:

1. It means that no external manifestations can exists (other than mechanical or chemical cause) without pre-existing altered internal dynamis.
2. However slight the external latent expression may appear, nevertheless the internal psora affects the whole organism, and any part or portion of the organism may sooner or later manifest it upon its surface.

Chapter 22

Bond of Psora with Life Forces[2]

Disease according to the orthodox school of medicine becomes a chemical accident, a dietetic error or microbial invasion; there is no primary vital principle.

The materialist would want us to believe that the physical, mental and moral expressions of life are dependent on chemistry. Ideas, thoughts, emotions, functions of organs, muscular contractions, loss or repair of tissue, physiological growth, that is the whole structural concept of human form, etiology, pathology, physiology, therapeutics all must conform to this chemical formula or bio-chemical model. Thus converting every organism into a laboratory for chemical purposes.

In the study of Psoric theory of disease we must not look from the bio-chemical side, but from Vital/ Potential side (Bio-physical side).

Psora is a potential that bonds itself with the life force (our inbuilt potential), that vital energy that not only animates the whole organism but sustains and controls all cell life and every physiological expression of life.

Psora is that potential which when becomes well bonded with the life force, it cooperates with this life force. Together these two along with other miasms, cause all physiological deflections, functional disturbances followed by structural and pathological changes.

The bond of the subversive forces with the life force is an invisible thing to be recognized only in its working with the life force, or in the new and strange phenomenon it presents as it perverts normal life action.

The nature and character of the disease depends wholly on the form of the miasm and the character of the bond with the life. Therefore the study of the disease becomes a study into the nature of miasm present in the organism and the degree of its activity.

Hahnemann's psoric theory of disease is the only true conception of disease. The new phenomena, or that which is supposed to be a new disease, is nothing more than the daily workings of miasm or the further development of miasm, a further expression of a perverted life action, a miasmatic revelation of that unknown dynamis, psora as seen in its pathological changes in the organism.

We know that behind every expression of life or matter there is an invisible dynamis. If this be true why not look for the dynamis for the pathological expression of disease? This is just what we should do.

The life force is that dynamis and the life force under normal conditions could not do other than give to that organism true physiological impulses and life sustaining qualities that is health.

Under the influence of perverted life action psora, life force is no longer a true dynamis but it is in bond with another dynamis, psora which knows no law and has no life giving qualities in it in fact all the dealings of psora are destructive.

The true internal nature of disease is thus made manifest in the study of the psoric theory of disease. Pathology can do nothing more for us today than it did in Hahnemann's time, for the simple reason that pathology is not at the bottom of that invisible process by which morbid changes and alterations take place in the organism.

What is said of the disease may be said of the potency. Although we see no material in potency, it still has the power to disturb the healthy organism in its own peculiar way.

It is the same with miasmatic potential; it is an invisible and unseen thing, yet we see the effects of its presence in the organism long before any changes of tissue take place. We see it first as a rule, first manifest in the mental sphere, then in the physiological or functional, then, finally, in the pathological, the pathological, of course, coming last.

Chapter 23

The Potential Study of Miasmatics[2]

We must always be on the lookout for the basic miasm in cases that do not yield to treatment. Nature always sets up; if possible, peripheral inhibitory points of disease, sometimes functional and often pathological in the sense that it tries to eliminate the products of degenerative processes.

If these inhibitory points are interfered locally without addressing the internal dynamic cause, the life force sets up another inhibitory center of reaction, nearer the deeper centers of life according to the law of progression and through the law of reaction.

A deeper inhibitory point can now no longer eliminate the products of degenerative processes in the life forces, set up by the more profound hold that the miasm has taken on the organism.

The vitality of the organism is slowly lowered so that now it has low resistive force or reactive power to set up another peripheral inhibition; therefore the organism succumbs to new order of changes of the now perverted life force.

The stress of the miasmatic force now centers upon new areas of the organism. The perverted physiological processes become more complex in their derangements or functions, and the retrograde metamorphosis (return of symptoms) becomes more difficult to analyze, until the therapeutist and the pathologist are so lost in the maze of symptomatology that they cannot systematically arrange or classify the symptoms.

It is in this way that advanced chronic diseases come, through a prolonged intoxication of the system, even to the remotest cell and fibers of being, due to pollution of life forces by some active miasm and if not remedied it will continue into a chronic form until every feature and outline of organism expresses symptomatic manifestation of their presence.

How generally we see the landmarks of one of these chronic miasms stamped upon the organism. We see it in every feature and every physiological process; in the shape and contour of the body; upon the visual expression; we see it on the skin; by the response in the very inner being, the mental, the moral, even the spiritual, give us responses of the presence and influence of miasm.

As we become more familiar with these subversive forces in their action upon the life force, or as we see their character expressed upon the normal vitality and function of the organism, how much more easy is it for us to follow their tracings or prophesy their probable development in any given case. If we become acquainted with the character of psora, whether expending its force upon the organism, simply, alone or in combination with some other miasm, we are more able to give a prognosis as to the probable outcome in a given case of disease; for the character and or combination of miasm gives us the character of disease or disease formula.

We see disease to be expression of three basic potential (pathophysiological trends). He who has become acquainted with the higher homoeopathics of Hahnemann, which comprises not only of disease potentials, but the drug action, can apply the law of similia at a deeper level.

As we study these miasm, we see they express themselves in their degrees of action (primary secondary and tertiary); and in their nature (acute, chronic and latent).

The bond of the subversive force with the life force is an invisible thing to be recognized only in its workings with the life force, or in the new and strange phenomena it presents as it hinders life action. The nature and character of the disease depends wholly on the form of the miasm and the character of the bond with the life; therefore the study of disease becomes a study into the:

1. Nature of the miasm present.
2. Degree of activity of miasm.

Chapter 24

Degree of Activity of Miasm[2,15]
(PRIMARY, SECONDARY & TERTIARY ACTION OF MIASM)

Primary action has no pathology it is functional and its realm of activity is mental and or vital. That which comes under the realm of pathology while the study of miasmatics is the secondary and tertiary manifestation of the miasm.

The first miasmatic potential is seen in the intoxication of the system long before the pathological appears this is the primary state of miasm.

The second miasmatic potential manifests in secondary skin eruption or discharge or ulcer this is the secondary action of the miasm.

The third potential is seen to partake when the secondary manifestations are suppressed and driven internally and the latent psora is aroused from its lethargy and intensifies and magnifies the action of both miasms producing tertiary manifestations of miasma.

Chapter 25

The Miasmatic Potential[2]

All life is magnified by continuous normal impulses from the great nerve centers of life such as brain. We see this dynamic potential in the power of speech, the action of the mind and yet overlook the dynamic potentiality of disease.

All these energies, all these potentials, are invisible, and when they finish their work on the organism we do not see the artist but a portrait.

It is the same dynamic potentiality that gives us these wonderful manifestations in life as in disease. In disease the life potential combines with the miasmatic potential.

The miasmatic potential is an invisible and unseen thing, yet we see the effects of its presence in the organism long before any tissue changes take place.

We see it first, as a rule, manifest in the mental sphere, then in the physiological or functional sphere and finally in the pathological, the pathological of course, coming last.

To many of us it is in this intervening space the mystery of disease lies. It is in this stage of the disease that the dynamis of the organism (the life force) is undergoing change or perversion- the intermingling of the false with the true, or the miasm with the life force, and the disturbances are in accordance with the existing active miasm, modified by previous heredity or miasmatic taint of the organism.

Herbert Spencer says, "We have no state of consciousness by which potential existence becomes actual". When we see in nature innumerable manifestation of these ever-present and ever acting invisible potential forces we say all actual material existence was first non-material potential existence.

Take for example action of growth by sunlight heat and moisture upon all life, stimulating, nourishing, developing, and showing that the actual is latent, dead, lifeless and undeveloped without the potential; therefore they are inseparable.

We have seen the relationship that the miasm bear to all diseases as a whole. We also saw their relation to functional disturbance and to pathology in general.

We have seen that all diseases were first disturbed function and that later on, as the functional disturbance increases and becomes more intensified, diseases became pathological. Indeed it is the perverted function or physiological stress that produces the pathological.

So we base the theory of all pathological formation and of every expression of pathology upon the grand truth that in all our dealings with matter, or the material, whether it be an organism or be it some inert medicinal substance or any therapeutic agent, we must deal with them from the potential side. To deal with them otherwise is to ignore the potential, to ignore the potential means to catalogue life with the material, with the chemical, and to raise it no higher than the chemical plane.

In the material or the actual plane it is the consciousness of form, of size, of color, etc. in the non-material or potential plane it is the consciousness of action, of change of position of motion.

It is this dynamic power that the miasm wield upon the life forces that we have to constantly deal with. It is through dynamic influences of miasm that all disease changes take place from the slightest functional disturbances to the most exaggerated pathological creations.

To us homoeopaths any pathological change or trend or formation is but a landmark of miasmatic action or change. They are simply ripening or ripened fruit of that prolonged perverted life action.

Let us now notice more closely this dual action of life force. The life force itself, in a normal state, is endowed with a creative power; but when we add to it the destructive action of some one or more of the miasms then we have a dual action set up.

To quote Spencer again "all vital action considered not separately but in wholeness have a purpose to balance certain outer process by certain inner processes". This balancing of the effects of force we call as equilibrium, and as soon as this barometer falls we have disease, and this prolonged dual action must sooner or later set up a counteraction, which gives us the inhibitory point. Therein a new and false action is set leading to a false and new creation (pathology).

In this way we can establish some true relation between what is seen - the real / material / pathological - and what is producing the pathological that is the invisible non-material phenomena, miasm.

We see then in abnormal physiological trends (pathology) two things: pathological condition and the phenomena of the condition. In the phenomena lies the cause of the pathological.

The phenomenon of appearance is not prima causa - rather it is the phenomenon of that invisible potens, psora, upon the life force.

Chapter 26

Inhibitory Points[2]

The father of all sickness, of whatever nature it may be, is directly or indirectly, a subversive force whose action is co-existence with the life force.

Through this mutually co-existence action we may have any conceivable anatomical, physiological or histological imperfection- moreover we may have a mental, moral or spiritual imperfection.

No lesion or pathological condition is the first cause of disease, for the disease process precedes them all, and the true cause always lies (other than mechanical) in the disturbed or distressed life force.

Let us try to understand the phenomena of inhibitory points by studying the genesis of tumor.

In the first place we must all admit that no abnormal growth can be formed without it being the work of life force. We will further admit that a normal or healthy life force could not and does not construct such growths, as it has no power other than it's normal physiologic action. Then how is a growth formed?

There are many ways by which the life force might be disturbed that would bring forth an abnormal growth, such as suppression of a discharge, injury to a part, suppression of disease states or any marked disease process. Any stasis of disease or miasmatic suppression may produce an abnormal growth.

Even should it be an hereditary expression the law holds good, because all abnormal growths are inhibitory points or inhibitory centers, and an inhibitory center is usually a tertiary expression of a miasm, although in acute cases it may be a secondary process.

When a miasm is acting along certain lines, say in chronic or sub acute state, producing simple external impressions, as papular eruptions, warts etc, the system is through these simple mediums eliminating from itself all the toxins generated by miasmatic pollution.

Should the unskilled physician who is not acquainted with this law governing miasmatics, suppresses these conditions, some other eliminating points must be created, as the miasm is still active in the organism with the same strength and power of action.

When we suppress the miasmatic action, the miasmatic force is directed against other lines and other points or parts in the organism. New phenomena and new symptoms develop. The more profound the suppression, the greater and deeper the new manifestation or new process.

Succeeding suppressions involves more vital center or organs, so that if we hit a single persistent symptom of a disease by specific medicines it is like breaking the tip of an iceberg.

So the physician without this knowledge hits with some specific remedy, or some suppressive measure every inhibitory point that manifests itself, and in that way he is constantly forcing every external manifestation of miasmatic action upon the organism itself, thus cutting of all avenues of elimination of the disease whose true nature he does not understand.

It is in this way abnormal growths develop, or that any new process develops which clinician classifies as new disease, independent, probably, of any former disease or state of the system.

We will now admit that abnormal growths come by or through this process of compelling the life forces along certain lines, due to combating a part of the phenomena of disease and not taking into consideration the totality of the phenomena.

We will now suppose that after we have done this thing we come to the true knowledge of disease

A tumor is but an inhibitory point due to perverted life action. It is a miasmatic correlating process.

A tumor, any abnormal growth for us homoeopaths is but a landmark of miasmatic action or change. We see in abnormal growths two things: the pathological condition and the phenomena of that condition. In the phenomena of that condition lays the cause of the pathological. We come to the conclusion that pathology is the creation of a life force perverted by miasmatic action, and that the phenomenon of appearance is not prima causa - rather it is the phenomenon of that invisible potens, psora.

Application of the law of similia to the active miasm is the only true method of curing the disease even when it has reached the pathological state.

We must look upon all disease, whether of a functional or pathological nature, from the potential side, and regard all phenomena as manifestations of some power within the organism itself.

The science of homoeopathy is correct grouping of all the relations' existing in the pathogenic phenomena of the life force, applying it to the law of similia, which is the shortest and most direct route to cure.

When the remedy thus chosen works we are encountered with a curative phenomenon called the retrograde metamorphosis.

In our study of retrograde process of disease many complex groupings of symptoms may present themselves for consideration and analysis, until perhaps a long history of perverted life action disappears in the reverse order in which it came.

The whole science of homoeopathy so far as therapeutics is concerned, becomes a study of the science of the forces and the law governing them, taking the true biological action of the life forces as a basis.

As the real or visible pathology came through the medium of the potential, or the perverted life action due to the miasms, so, in the like manner, it disappears through the potential by virtue of the power and by the assistance of another potential, the similimum of homoeopathic potency. This is the true healing and is embraced in the teachings of the first paragraph of the organon.

This conflict between the life force and the miasms furnishes us, as healers of the sick, with the material for a life study, along with all the ills, with all the phenomena, subjective and objective, visible and invisible, that fills our works on practice and our volumes on therapeutics, with data of the phenomena of disturbed vital force.

In the beginning of this miasmatic conflict, or when the miasm are in latent condition, we see only flag signs of distress, only threatening of greater future distress, as seen in wandering pains or the mild sensations of heat and cold etc. Then we may see great centers profoundly disturbed, as in epilepsy, spasm, convulsions, until we get any degree of pathology.

A nebulous of disease is but a nebulous of perverted motion, and a climax of disease is a climax of action in perverted life force. We live or exist on a higher plane of action, even as the life forces act upon a higher or lower plane. It is the momentum that kills or makes alive; forces must be magnified or diminished before lines of action are changed or destroyed.

We are compelled to confine ourselves to the study of the phenomena, the nature of which confirms the kind of bond the subversive force has made with the life force. When this bond proves to be inseparable we call the disease incurable, and when it can be separated, curable. The persistency of the bond establishes the relationship between the life forces and the subversive forces.

If the balance of power is on the side of the life force the subversive force is latent. But if the balance of power were on the side of the subversive force, then we look at any degree of intensity or persistence of disease. This is as true of the functional as it is of a simple pathological state.

Thus we have found that the real, the actual, is but the creation of the potential; that the real has no existence but through the potential; that the correlation of the forces is behind all things, and if we wish to know or to see what disease is we must know and see it through the potential. If we would remove disease from the suffering organism we must remove it in like manner - that is, by and through the potency of medicine.

We will now suppose that after we have done and understood all this thing we come to the true knowledge of disease and the desire to undo the work performed by miasmatic force. How shall we do it?

There is but one way, and that is by taking carefully the present existing totality, which uncovers the cause and establishes a retrograde metamorphosis.

By taking carefully this new totality groupings in order of their appearance we are led to the primary simple miasmatic state and in the meantime the pathology is removed and along with that are removed all the sufferings that we call a disease.

In the first place, as we study this totality, our knowledge of its grouping tells us to what miasm it belongs. In retrograde metamorphosis of abnormal growth or any such complex disease we are encountered with symptom groupings of miasma succeeding each other, these form the basis of layered approach of homoeotherapeutics.

If we happen to be orthodox medical clinician our first anxiety is to know what is the origin of the growth (histo-pathological classification) and its grade (TNM Classification); knowing that greatly modifies our prognosis and possibility of cure. Yet to know this (histological origin) does not lead us back fully to the cause, as the histo-pathological process is not prima causa, because we homoeopaths know that certain miasm originally produced this condition.

In order to get at the basic principles of a neoplastic process we must investigate its miasmatic origin. But critics will say how do you know that a miasm is behind or at the root of all abnormal growths?

We know following the Hahnemannian thought, experiment and analysis that miasm lay not only at the basis of abnormal growths but that they fathered all disease other than chemical and mechanical irritation.

In the second place, when the law of cure is applied basing the prescription on the totality of the prominent and most dependent miasmatic symptoms, the abnormal growth no longer develops and if the case is not far advanced these growths begin to regress and resolve.

This occurs when highest potencies are given (in high potencies all the chemical action is lost in preparing the remedy by process of potentization).

In selecting the similar remedy the local symptoms or pathological phenomena is either not taken into consideration or is only given its due place in anamnesis of the case.

It is evident with the response we get from homoeopathic medicine that the abnormal growth looses its power to increase in size and begins to diminish, and furthermore that the general health of the patient begins to improve immediately with the arrest of growth. This is sufficient proof of the basic principle lying at the bottom of the disease has been reached; besides no other drug induced or otherwise new disease process develops.

On the other hand if the growth is removed by surgical measures, it often either becomes recurrent, or some new development succeeds it, frequently of a nervous or mental nature, which is difficult to cure.

So we see that the removal of tumor by surgical measure is simply the removal of this inhibitory center, which the life forces were compelled to set up, owing to perverted life motion. When this miasmatically correlative point is surgically excised we see some other organ where the disease phenomena settles.

What further verification do we need to prove that the basic principle of disease is potential. In looking upon the disease from this standpoint we readily see that reality underlies appearances as the law of similia unfolds the mystery of prima causa.

The process of resolution taking place in any abnormal growth, under the law of similia, through the influence of a potency, is nothing more than a cessation of miasmatic action and the retrograde metamorphosis of the life force resuming its normal again, and as we analyze perverted life action as a whole it leads us back not only to cause but to a true conclusion of the unknown- it finds the secret power, the miasm, that is behind the perversion and the homoeopathic potency neutralizes miasmatic action and annuls its power over the organism.

Chapter 27

The Nature of Miasm[2,15,16] Latent & Chronic

Perverted life force, under the influence of invisible subversive force psora lies slumbering so to say in the invisible interiors of an organism and it was named as latent psora by Hahnemann.

When the miasmatic forces lie dormant in the organism, the organism appears to be healthy. Hahnemann himself gave us a list of symptoms that give us a clue of latent psora.

Suffering from several or front a greater number of these ailments [even at various times and frequently], a person will still consider himself as healthy, and is supposed to be so by others. With such persons the psora [internal itch malady], which may be recognized by a connoisseur by means of a few or by more of the above symptoms, may slumber on for many years within, without causing any continuing chronic disease.

But still, even in such favorable external relations, as soon as these persons advance in age, even moderate causes [a slight vexation, or a cold, or an error in diet, etc.], may produce a violent attack of [however only a brief] disease: a violent attack of colic, inflammation of the chest or the throat, erysipelas, fever and the like, and the violence of these attacks seems to be out of proportion to its moderate cause. This is mostly wont to happen in fall or winter, but often also by preference in springtime.

In a similar manner, a robust merchant, apparently healthy, despite some traces of internal Psora, perceptible only to the professional examiner, may in consequence of unlucky commercial conjunctures become involved in his finances, even so as to approach bankruptcy, and at the same time he will fall gradually into various ailments and finally into serious illness. The death of a rich kinsman, however, and the gaining of a great prize in a lottery, abundantly cover his commercial losses; he becomes a man of means-but his illness, nevertheless, not only continues but increases from year to year, despite all medical prescriptions, in spite of his visiting the most famous baths, or rather, perhaps, with the assistance of these two causes.

A modest girl, who, excepting some signs of internal psora, was accounted quite healthy, was compelled into a marriage which made her unhappy of soul, and in the same degree her bodily health declined, without any trace of venereal infection. No allopathic medicine alleviates her sad ailments, which continually grow more threatening. But in the midst of this aggravation, after one year's suffering, the cause of her unhappiness, her hated husband, is taken from her by death, and she seems to revive, in the conviction, that she is now delivered from every occasion of mental or bodily illness, and hopes for a speedy recovery; all her friends hope the same for her, as the exciting cause of her illness lies in the grave. She also improves speedily, but unexpectedly she still remained an invalid, despite the vigor of her youth; yea, her ailments but seldom leave her, and are renewed from time to time without any external cause, and they are even aggravated·from year to year in the rough months.

A person who had been unjustly suspected and become involved in a serious criminal suit, and who bad before seemed healthy, with the exception of the marks of latent psora mentioned below, during these harassing months fell into various diseased states. But finally the innocence of the accused is acknowledged, and an honorable acquittal followed. We might suppose that such a happy, gratifying event would necessarily give new life to the accused and remove all bodily complaints. But this does not take place, the person still at times suffers from these ailments, and they are even renewed with longer or brief intermissions, and are aggravated with the passing years, especially in-the winter seasons.

How shall we explain this? If that disagreeable event had been the cause, the sufficient cause, of these ailments, ought not the effect; i.e., the disease, to have entirely ceased of necessity, after the removal of the cause? But these ailments do not cease, they are in time renewed and even gradually aggravated, and it becomes evident that those disagreeable events could not have been the sufficient cause of the present ailments and complaints. It is seen that they only served as an occasion and impetus toward the development of a malady, which till then only slumbered within.

The recognition of this old internal foe, which is so frequently present, and the science which is able to overcome it, make it manifest, that generally an indwelling itch disease [psora] was the ground of all these ailments, which can not be overcome even by the vigor of the best constitution, but only through art.

The awakening of the internal psora which has hitherto slumbered and been latent, and, as it were, kept bound by a good bodily constitution and favorable external circumstances, as well as its breaking out into more serious ailments and maladies, is announced by the increase of the symptoms given above as indicating the slumbering psora, and also by a numberless multitude of various other signs and complaints. These are varied according to the difference in the bodily constitution of a man, his hereditary disposition, the various errors in his education and habits, his manner of living and diet, his employments, his turn of mind, his morality, etc.

LATENT MIASM[15]

Perverted life force, under the influence of invisible subversive force psora lies slumbering so to say in the invisible interiors of an organism and it was named as latent psora by Hahnemann. When the miasmatic forces lie dormant in the organism, the organism appears to be healthy. Hahnemann himself gave us a list of symptoms that give us a clue of latent psora.

SYMPTOMS OF LATENT PSORA IN CHILDREN

1. Frequent discharge of *Ascaris* and other worms; intolerable itching caused by the latter in the rectum.
2. The abdomen often distended.
3. Now insatiable hunger, then again want of appetite.
4. Paleness of the face and relaxation of the muscles.
5. Frequent inflammations of the eyes.
6. Swellings of the cervical glands [scrofula].
7. Perspiration on the head, in the evening after going to sleep.

SYMPTOMS OF LATENT PSORA IN ADULTS

1. Epistaxis in girls and youths [more rarely with older persons], often very severe.
2. Usually cold hands or perspiration on the palms, [burning in the palms].
3. Cold, dry, or ill-smelling sweaty feet, [burning in the soles of the feet].
4. The arms or hands, the legs or feet, are benumbed by a slight cause.
5. Frequent cramps in the calves [the muscles of the arms and hands].

6. Painless subsultus (lipoma) of various portions of the muscles here and there on the body.
7. Frequent or tedious dry or fluent coryza or catarrh or impossibility of catching a cold even from the most severe exposure, even While otherwise having-continually ailments of this kind.
8. Long continued obstruction of one or both nostrils.
9. Ulcerated nostrils [sore nose].
10. Disagreeable sensation of dryness in the nose.
11. Frequent inflammation of the throat, frequent hoarseness.
12. Short cough in the morning.
13. Frequent attacks of dyspnoea.
14. Predisposition to catching cold (The epidemic catarrhal fevers and catarrhs which seize almost, everyone, even the healthiest persons [Grippe, influenza], do not belong to this category.)
15. Predisposition to sprains, even from carrying or lifting a slight weight, [so also a multitude of complaints resulting from a moderate stretching of the muscles: headache, nausea, prostration, tensive pain in the muscles of the neck and back, etc.]
16. Frequent one-sided headache or toothache, even from moderate emotional disturbances.
17. Frequent flushes of heat and redness of the face, not infrequently with anxiety.
18. Frequent falling out of hair of the head, dryness of the same, and many scales upon the scalp.
19. Predisposition to erysipelas now and then.
20. Amenorrhoea, irregularities in the menses, too copious, too scanty, too early [too late], of too long duration, too watery, connected with various bodily ailments.

21. Twitching of the limbs on going to sleep.
22. Weariness early on awaking; unrefreshing sleep.
23. Perspiration in the morning in bed.
24. Perspiration breaks out too easily during the daytime, even with little movement [or inability to bring out perspiration].
25. White, or at least very pale tongue; still more frequently cracked tongue.
26. Much phlegm in the throat.
27. Bad smell from the mouth, Sour taste in the mouth, dryness in the mouth.
28. Nausea, in the morning.
29. Sensation of emptiness in the stomach.
30. Repugnance to cooked, warm food, especially to meat [principally with children].
31. Repugnance to milk.
32. Cutting pains in the abdomen, frequently or daily [especially with children].
33. Hard stools, often covered with mucus
34. Venous knots on the anus; passage of blood with the stools.
35. Passing of mucus from the anus, with or without faeces.
36. Dark urine.
37. Swollen, enlarged veins on the legs [swollen veins, varices].
38. Chilblains
39. Pains as of corns, without any external pinching of the shoes.
40. Disposition to crack, strain or wrench one joint or another.
41. Cracking of one or more joints on moving.
42. Renewal of pains and complaints while at rest, and disappearance of the same while in motion.

43. Most of the ailments come on at night, and are increased with a low barometer, with north and northeast winds, in winter and towards spring.
44. Uneasy, frightful, or at least too vivid, dreams.
45. Unhealthy skin; every little lesion passes into sores; cracked skin of the hands and of the lower lips.
46. Frequent boils, frequent felons [whitlows].
47. Dry skin on the limbs; on the arms, the thighs, and also at times on the cheeks.
48. Here or there a rough, scaling spot on the skin, which causes at times a voluptuous itching and, after the rubbing, a burning sensation.
49. Here or there at times, though seldom, a single insufferably pleasant, but unbearably itching vesicle, at its point sometimes filled with pus, and causing a burning sensation after rubbing, on a finger, on the wrist or in some other place.

Suffering from several or front a greater number of these ailments [even at various times and frequently], a person will still consider himself as healthy, and is supposed to be so by others. With such persons the psora [internal itch malady], which may be recognized by a connoisseur by means of a few or by more of the above symptoms, may slumber on for many years within, without causing any continuing chronic disease.

SECTION V: MIASMA AS DISEASE CAUSATIVE FORCE

Chapter 28

Inquiry into the Process of Disease Phenomenon

Chapter 29

Hahnemann's Causative Classification of Disease

Chapter 30

Suppression of Miasma

Chapter 31

The Eizayaga Model of Layers of Disease

Chapter 32

How to Recognize Miasma by Symptoms

Chapter 33

Key Characteristics of Miasma

Chapter 28

Inquiry into the Process[8,9] of Disease Phenomenon

When I call disease a derangement of man's state of health, I am far from wishing thereby to give a hyperphysical explanation of the internal nature of diseases generally, or of any case of disease in particular.

It is only intended by this expression to intimate, what it can be proved disease are not and cannot be, that they are not mechanical or chemical alteration of the material substance of the body, and not dependent on a material morbific substance, but that they are merely spiritual dynamic derangements of the life.

Footnote § 31

The inimical forces, partly psychical, partly physical, to which our terrestrial existence is exposed, which are termed morbific noxious agents, do are not possess the power of morbidly deranging the health of man unconditionally.

We are made ill by them only when our organism is sufficiently disposed and susceptible to the attack of the morbific cause that may be present, hence they do not produce disease in every one nor at all times.

Incalculably greater and more important than the two chronic miasms just named, however, it is the chronic miasm of psora, which, whilst those two reveal their specific internal dyscracia, the one by the venereal chance, the other by the cauliflower-like growths, does also, after the completion of the internal infection of the whole organism, announce by a peculiar cutaneous eruption, sometimes consisting only of a few vesicles accompanied by intolerable voluptuous tickling itching (and a peculiar odor), the monstrous internal chronic miasm the psora.

Psora is the only real fundamental cause and producer of all the other numerous, I may say innumerable, forms of disease, which, under the names of nervous debility, hysteria, hypochondriasis, mania, melancholia, imbecility, madness, epilepsy and convulsions of all sorts, softening of the bones (rachitis), scoliosis and kyphosis, caries, cancer, fungus haematodes, neoplasms, gout, haemorrhoids, jaundice, cyanosis, dropsy, amenorrhoea, hemorrhage from the stomach, nose, lungs, bladder and womb, of asthma and ulceration of the lungs, of impotence and barrenness, of megrim, deafness, cataract, amaurosis, urinary calculus, paralysis, defects of the senses and pains of thousands of kinds, &c., figure in systematic works on pathology as peculiar, independent diseases.

§ 80

During the flourishing years of youth and with the commencement of regular menstruation joined to a mode of life beneficial to soul, heart and body, psora remains unrecognized for years, Those afflicted appear in perfect health to their relative and acquaintances and the disease that was received by infection or inheritance seems to have wholly disappeared.

In later years, after adverse events and conditions of life, they are sure to appear a fresh and develop the more rapidly and assume a more serious character in proportion as the vital principle has become disturbed by debilitating passions, worry and care, but especially when disordered by inappropriate medicinal treatment.

§ 78 (Sixth Edition)

If we deduct all chronic affections, ailments and disease that depend on a persistent unhealthy mode of living (§ 77), as also those innumerable medicinal maladies (§ 74) caused by the irrational persistent, harassing and pernicious treatment of disease often only of trivial character by physicians of the old school, all the remainder, [chronic diseases], without exception, result from the development of these three chronic miasms, internal syphilis, internal sycosis, but chiefly and in infinitely greater proportion, internal psora, each of which was already in possession of the whole organism, and had penetrated it in all directions before the appearance of the primary, vicarious local symptom of each of them.

These chronic miasmatic disease are inevitably destined by mighty nature sooner or later to become, develop and to burst forth and thereby propagate all the nameless misery, the incredible number of chronic disease which have plagued mankind for hundreds and thousands of years, these three miasms can be radically by the internal homoeopathic medicines suited for each of them, without employing topical remedies for their external symptoms.

§ 204

It is evident that man's vital force, when encumbered with a chronic disease is unable to overcome by its own powers [Instinctively] adopts the plan of developing local malady on some external part, solely for this object, it chooses by making and keeping a diseased state in the part which is not indispensable to human life, it may thereby silence the internal disease, which otherwise threatens to destroy the vital organs, and that it may thereby, so to speak, transfer the internal disease to the vicarious local affection thus silences, for a time, the internal disease, though without being able either to cure it or to diminish it materially.

The local affection, however, is never anything else than a part of the general internal disease, but a part of it increased only in one direction by the organic vital force, and transferred to a less dangerous (external) part of the body, in order to allay the internal ailment.

The internal disease, on the contrary, continues, in spite of it, gradually to increase and Nature is constrained to enlarge and aggravate the local symptom always more and more, in order that it may still suffice as a substitute for the increased internal disease and may still keep it under. Old ulcers on the legs get worse as long as the internal syphilis remains uncured, the fig warts increase and grow while the sycosis in not cured whereby the latter is rendered more and more difficult to cure, just as the general internal disease continues to increase as time goes on.

§ 201

Among chronic diseases we must still, alas! reckon those so, artificially produced by allopathic treatment and by the prolonged use of violent heroic medicines in large and increasing doses, by whereby the vital force is sometimes weakened to an unmerciful extent, sometimes, if it do not succumb, gradually abnormally deranged (by each substance in a peculiar manner).

In order to maintain life against these inimical and destructive attacks, it must produce a revolution in the organism, and either deprive some part of its irritability and sensibility, or exalt these to an excessive degree, cause dilatation or contraction, relaxation or induration or even total destruction or certain parts, and develop faulty organic alterations here and there in the interior or the exterior in order to preserve the organism from complete destruction of life by the ever-renewed, hostile assaults of such destructive forces.

§ 74

In these paragraphs of the Organon of the medicine Hahnemann is describing what we now call natural history of a chronic disease. In the chronic disease. Pg. 39-97 Hahnemann describes stage of development of any chronic disease. i.e. the natural history of a chronic disease.

- Inception of Disease (§ 80)
- Development of Disease (footnote § 78)
- Appearance of primary symptoms (§ 201)
- Appearance of secondary symptoms (§ 74)

§ 31 is nothing else but a concept of man amidst disease.

In § 204 Hahnemann describes about multifactorial causation of disease.

Chapter 29

Hahnemann's Causative[25] Classification of Disease

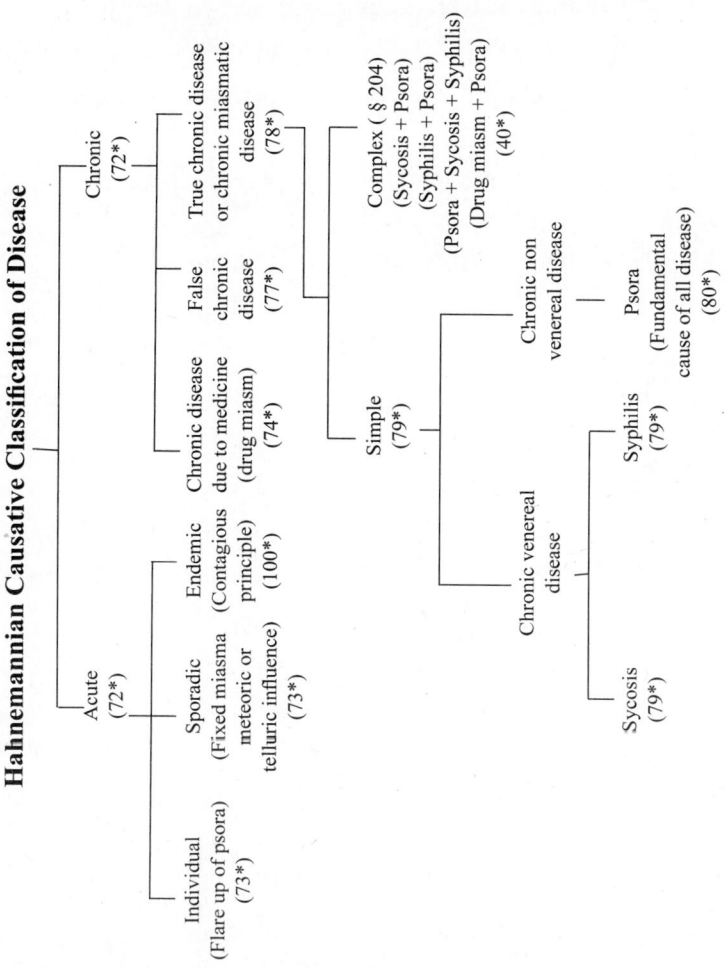

Figure 12: Hahnemann's Causative Classification of Disease

Chapter 30

Suppression of Miasma[2,5,7,13,15,20,21,26,28,37,50]

Hahnemann, speaking of the treatment of psora in his Chronic Diseases, Vol. 1, says: "The older physicians were much more conscientious than modern doctors, they were much more enlightened observers. Their practice was based upon experience, which showed them that the removal of psoric eruption from the skin was followed by innumerable ailments and grievous maladies."

However true this may be, today we have reason to believe that they saw in the psoric eruption an internal constitutional disease and attempted, in their weak and very imperfect way, to treat it constitutionally, and not locally. It is true that thousands of practitioners today recognize psora, and all the chronic miasms, for that matter, as internal constitutional affections. But, not knowing the methods which Hahnemann employed, or not being acquainted with a law of cure, they can not apply internal medicines in a way that will remove their effects from the organism; therefore, not knowing what else to do, they resort to expedients of all kinds, not as a matter of choice, but from that of necessity.

The majority of men are honest in these things, and would gladly adopt our methods if they understood them; but they are so diverse and so different from the teachings of the scientists of today that in order to change their methods of treatment they would, to a great degree, have to abandon or cast aside their present teachings and knowledge of physiology and pathology in general; even their conception of life, as well as therapeutics, must be changed.

They would have to put a dynamic life force behind their physiology and abandon their theory of chemical action as governing the growth and repair of the organism, and accept Hahnemann's dynamic theory of both disease and life. Thus you see some of the reasons why men use expedients and all sorts of methods in the treatment of the sick. And what are they contending against? Disease they call it.

They have endeavored to tabulate and give a special name to each miasmatic expression present in the organism, but often the name itself is confusing, and misleading; old names are retained such as rheumatism, and many others we might mention which were conceived in ignorance and framed from a misconception not only of life, but of disease. New names are today coined with almost as poor a conception of their origin or their nature.

Often-the organ or part affected is coupled with changes that are apparent or which really take place in the medical circulation. Again the character of the lesion is coupled with the organ or affected part and thus the disease manifestation receives its permanent name; with this name they are compelled to place a pathological or etiological explanation, in order that it may be understood.

You see such a state of things exist because men do not understand the causus morbii, the miasms, which are the true etiological factors in disease, which are to be studied carefully in order to understand the relationship to disease, whether functional or pathological.

These multiple expressions of disease, known by certain specified names, are but the fruits of the miasmatic action and its power in our study of disease we over function and over life may lose sight of the miasm itself for a time, as it becomes more or less latent in the organism or is presented in new forms and as new phenomena, but we can never lose sight of that force, that unknown quantity, which is constantly perverting the life and bringing changes in the organism, and although we may not recognize it as one of the chronic miasms, it nevertheless is, and if we bring the life forces under law we at the same time bring it under law, "that is the miasm".

Now if we bring the life force under law we have brought all under law, and we can have no suppression. Should we, however, not recognize either law, life force, or miasm, we are forced to go back to chemical medicine, and to our empirical measures, and the life force must suffer the consequences and become more and more deflected until pathological states and conditions arise without name and without number.

We can only understand the forces of nature by and through law; because law is reveal all things, as it is only through it that this unknown principle (the miasm) is clearly revealed to us with all its attending phenomena.

It is also true that we can only see through law the mystery of a suppression, for suppression itself is a retrograde process or a deflection of law, or it is physiological law opposed.

The physician who suppresses any miasmatic state, or disease process, if you wish, is an enemy of law, or at least there is no mutual understanding between him and law.

We must first know that law rules not alone the visible things, but all invisible as well. It stops not at potency, but governs all the forces, and in disease there is no exception.

You may ask the question, shall we give any consideration to apply our medicines locally? No. I say most emphatically-no, as that is not according to any law of life, or disease for that matter.

Why? Because you know disease is perverted life force from within outward, and from above downward, and not from without inward. The life is within, not without; the disease is within, not upon the surface. It is only an expression of it that you see. You can never see disease, any more than you can see life itself.

If it were possible for it to be visible it could not bond with the life force, and this fact is true in every expression and every phase of homoeopathy; to withdraw from this is to withdraw from homoeopathy, as thousands have done, leaving only the name behind them as a memorial, although that name is by no means represented in its true light.

"Life," says Hahnemann, "is a vital principle, a self-moving force, a vital power which, if acting in harmony, preserves our bodies a harmonious whole; a disturbance of which is disease; a lack of which is death".

Herbert Spencer says, "Life is a continuous adjustment of internal relations to external". It is by virtue of this fact we are entitled to be called alive. True, we are constantly adjusting ourselves to changes, so that any altered condition in our life force throws us out of harmony.

The adjustment is always imperfect in the presence of the miasm, and it is this imperfect adjustment with which we are constantly dealing in chronic miasmatic disease. The external adjustment is imperfect only when the internal is imperfect in chronic miasmatic disease. It is the internal, the life, that rules the organism. When it is perfect the organism is perfect, and when it is imperfect the organism is more or less imperfect.

So, we see that the life harmony dwells in the law. If disease is internal, we can not assist it from without. Therapeutically speaking, then, we must enter into correspondence with it, we must deal with that which animates the organism and gives it its being, the life. Nature is the complement of the life; but we must assist nature through its right channels and by the way of law. Disease appears through the medium of the same law that governs life, and we must work with it along these lines.

The life force often relieves itself from the possibility of a suppression due to our treatment by presenting the existing miasmatic action in some new form or by an external expression, for instance, in an eruptive disease, in a diarrhea, in a neuralgia.

Thus the outward expression must relieve the inward expression. Death follows when these conditions are not equalized. And that is what is meant by equilibrium, which is the balancing of the effects of force or the effects of the miasm upon the perverted life force.

HOW SUPPRESSION MAY TAKE PLACE

Hahnemann in his Chronic Diseases, Vol. 1, devotes seventeen or eighteen pages to the subject of suppression, wherein he gives special cases illustrating almost every form of suppression and the means whereby they are produced. He puts particular stress upon the suppression of skin eruptions, such as itch (scabies), tenia, eczema and other such eruptive diseases.

Out of which arise some of the most fatal results, or which may be the means of establishing new disease processes which are even more dangerous to life or are more difficult to eradicate.

The most frequent methods used to suppress were local applications, such as itch ointments, salves, medicated lotions, mineral baths, applications of cold and heat, also the persistent use of crude drugs internally.

The same author says that the removal of the local expression of the disease only gave the miasm an opportunity to become centralized upon some organ of the body and that while the local expressions were removed the internal conditions were unchanged, and the internal disease increased in the progress of time.

He recognized the local symptoms as secondary expressions, or vicarious expressions of the internal disorder. He also noticed that the suffering of the organism was greatly relieved when the patient broke out with an eruption or when any external manifestations of disease presented themselves, whether they were skin eruptions, catarrhal discharges, diarrhea, dysuria, hemorrhoids, abnormal growths or any other local manifestations.

He further noticed that with these sufferings and attended with these comings and goings of the disease or these inward and outward miasmatic manifestations, the internal suffering either ceased entirely or was greatly relieved as the local expressions presented themselves, such as eruptions, perspirations, abscesses, discharges and so on. It was such expressions that enabled him to see the true nature and character of disease, which he followed to its bond with the life force itself and from which all disease emanated.

While the local methods of treating skin eruptions, ulcers and local lesions is still in vogue they are not so generally used at the present time as they have been then. However, still more powerful agents are now in use which not only accomplish the same purpose but do it more effectively and with more certainty. A few of these I will mention, such as the actual cautery, so largely in use to destroy chancroid ulcerations and other ulcerations where bacteria are supposed to be abundantly present.

When we suppress any local disease we overcome that process or we annul it, and we are then enemies physiological law. This is the secret of all suppression we have deflected, nature's eliminative process, which is a life process, and have forced nature and its processes back upon itself.

We must not lose sight of the fact that while we are dealing with disease we are dealing with life, "for all disease processes are perverted life processes," and all must be brought under the laws of life in order to restore that disturbed harmony.

If we study closely we will see that it is the same law that governs all life. It is biological law governing; not chemistry, but biological dynamics.

As we rise in the scale of life and begin to deal with multicellular forms and biotic life as a whole, when organs and life processes are multiplied, then we get that multiplicity of phenomena which makes it the more difficult to analyze and harder to understand.

We might illustrate this, in a way, by taking into account the child at puberty, when the reproductive processes are developing. Previous to this we had not this sphere to deal with, and if at all, only to a very slight degree. But now we have a very complex process that is subject to numberless changes and disease processes.

So we see, as organs are added, the life process becomes more complete, therefore the disease processes are more numerous and complex. Again, as the miasms are multiplied the disease processes become still more complex and multiplied, so that the effects of a suppression is then more complex in its phenomena, therefore more dangerous to life.

If we suppress psora we are aware of the profound changes which take place in that organism from a simple pruritis to pain, spasm, convulsions, coma, and death. But when we suppress a mixed miasm, like psora and sycosis, what can we expect? We certainly must expect multiple processes and fearful conditions to follow; for the character of each, subversive force, each miasm will be characterized and, to some degree, expressed in that organism.

If we deal with disease from any other standpoint, we can not give it the positive assistance we would like in each disease state and prevent all danger of suppression or deflexion of the miasms action.

The suppressed action of a chronic miasm means much to the patient, to the family and to the race in general, for it not only weakens the race, but it means (as a rule) hereditary transmission of either that, perverted state, or that deeper and more profound, involvement, by these newly developed processes, coming out of such suppressions.

There is another point to be considered in our study of the suppression of the miasms and that is the resistive power of the life force. One person is gifted with more power than another; different persons resist to a greater or less degree the action of drugs. One patient is sensitive to a certain drug or remedy; another one is comparatively insensitive. A local application of a certain crude drug applied to certain eruptive diseases readily dissipates it in one patient, while it has comparatively no effect upon another, and vice versa.

This may be due to some idiosyncrasy in the patient or it may be due to some natural protective or resistive force in the organism or hereditary.

I have often noticed that when many crude drugs, now in use for the suppression of some local manifestation of disease, fail to accomplish the result, some other means has to be used to accomplish the work. Again, often when disease is suppressed, it will not remain so, but will be forever breaking forth, either in the same form and in the same locality, or in similar form and in different localities.

In this way the life force largely protects itself against the inroads of this unscientific and inaccurate method of combating disease. Again the organism may be gifted with that inherent power to set up other local manifestations of miasmatic action, such as pain, neuralgia, rheumatism and such kindred diseases, which will largely take the place of primary eruptive diseases, and in that way prevent an internal miasmatic stasis.

If we attempt to suppress the disease locally by local measures, in a patient with very little resistive force, or where the resistive power of the life force is below par, or where they have been under the effects for a long time of some mixed miasm, such as tuberculosis, the suppression is often an easy matter; but where we attempt to suppress disease in some strong, vigorous constitution the life force rebels and the contest becomes a marked one between the therapeutic agent and the life force.

All the principles of life governing the organism are principles of truth, and when any of them are interfered with nature rebels. This protective principle.

The life force before the attempt at suppression was either eliminating, or endeavoring to eliminate all miasmatic products, or that produced by the disease process, which is in agreement with physiological law.

The false physician, the violator of law comes in and opposes it, turning it about, and thus magnifies the disease process, by forcing a change of action, or some new process of disease upon the organism.

In that way, not only is the disease changed, but the symptomatology is changed and as we attempt now to take the case, we get an imperfect picture of the true internal change due to the deflection, and besides only a part of the symptomatology is presented and that is in an imperfect light, and the rest is veiled or covered from our sight. Herein is the point where disease is made incurable.

AN UPDATED ACCOUNT ON SUPPRESSION OF DISEASE

WHAT IS INTERNAL DISORDER?

We must clearly perceive what do we understand by interior this could be understood by Nigam's layers & levels of human forms which is

THE LAYERS OF HUMAN FORM

From External to Internal

1. Human Body = The Material Plane = The Body Matrix = Outermost Layer 1
2. Vital Force = The Lower Dynamic Plane = The Dynamis = Layer 2
3. Central Controlling Axis = Layer 3 (comprises of Central; Autonomic; Peripheral Nervous Systems and also the endocrine glands)
4. Mind = The Higher Dynamic Plane = Layer 4
5. Soul = The Virtual Plane = Layer 5

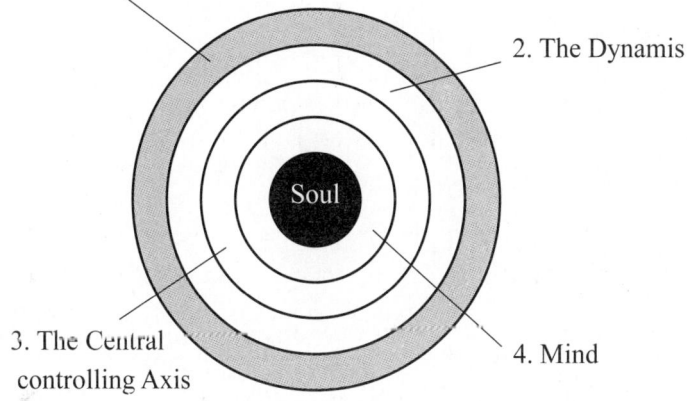

Figure 13: Layers of Human Form

The organism is indeed the material instrument of life but it is not conceivable without the animation imparted to it by the innately perceiving and regulating dynamis, just as the dynamis is not conceivable without the organism consequently the two together constitute a unity although in thought our mind separates this unity into two distinct conceptions for the sake of easy comprehension

Hahnemann. S. Aphorism 15; The Organon of Medical Art

In Homoeopathy we are particularly concerned with the dynamic plane. This dynamic energy Hahnemann discerned as two the mind and the vital force (wesen). Hahnemann saw in the body but an organism made up of material particles by themselves dead, but vivified embodied and adapted to the real, living man, the spirit within. The connection between mind and the body is supposed by him to be effected by means of the vital force which he designates Dynamis.

We have then in Hahnemannian physiology:

1. The spirit, the true man, the mind.
2. The vivifying vital force, the Dynamis, maintaining the life and health.
3. The material body.

The inner dynamic plane of Mind, the outer dynamic plane of vital force. The inner dynamic plane vivifies the central controlling axis while the outer dynamic plane of vital force maintains the material plane of human body.

From these conception follows the deduction that the disturbance of the harmonious play of life, manifesting itself in symptoms affecting the functions and sensations, which we call disease, is a disturbance of this vital force (Aphorism 11). This vital force is in fact the inner force, which controls the molecular, chemical and mechanical processes, and uses them for its own purpose of self-preservation. The vital force is the intermediate agent between the mind and the body, enabling the mind to control the material body.

This layered concept will help you to understand that the Hahnemannian concept of the internal origin of disease.

It is to be understood clearly that according to Hahnemann in most cases the internal disorder is first in the vital plane i.e. the layer of dynamis [Aphorism 11; 12; 72]. In such cases of we find alteration both in mind (mental Symptoms) and in the material body (somatic symptoms) [Aphorism 210 & Aphorism 214]. Hahnemann also says that in some cases the internal disorder starts from the mind and eventually ruins the material body [Aphorism 225]. This is the only value of understanding the Nigam's layered concept of human form & the reader should refer to the simplified concept of human form by the author for detailed study of these concepts.

Now we move to what are the Planes of human forms. This was a concept first proposed by Kent. French Homoeopaths further enhanced it. What I present is the modified version of French concept. This is a vital concept to understand because this would help the homoeopath to understand: The Planes of Internal Disorder, The Hering's law, The Theory of Suppression and the basis of the selection of Potency.

THE LAYERS OF HUMAN EXISTENCE	THE PLANES OF HUMAN EXISTENCE
THE MIND	THE PLANE OF MIND
THE DYNAMIS/VITAL	THE PLANE OF DYNAMIS/ VITAL FORCE
THE CENTRAL CONTROLLING AXIS	CNS
	ANS
	ENDOCRINE
THE BODY MATRIX	HUMORAL
	VISCERAL
	MECHANICAL
	SKIN

Figure 14: Layers of Human Form

This concept clarifies that there are two levels of internal disorders

The dynamic imbalances are

1. Psychological = The plane of sickness is at the mental plane.
2. Miasmatic (non-chromosomal inherited traits) = The plane of sickness is mental & the plane of dynamis.
3. Constitutional (Multifactorial/Multifaceted) that is all the above three along with organic pathology.

The imbalance at the material plane can be

1. Hereditary (Inherited via chromosomes) = The plane of sickness is the material body.
2. Immunological = The plane of sickness is Humoral
3. Organic Pathology = The plane of sickness is Visceral/Mechanical/skin plane.

WHAT IS SUPPRESSION?

- The exterior/peripheral symptoms, when removed without addressing the underlying dynamic cause can lead to internal systemic disease.
- Thus the progression of disease due to suppression is

1. From external to within.
2. From less vital to more vital parts.

An account of Suppression of symptoms & skin disease is given in Para 187-203 of The Organon & Chapter Psora of The Chronic Diseases, The gist of which has been illustrated in the previous chapter. Along with a detailed account by H.C. Allen.

ENQUIRY INTO THE PHENOMENON OF CHRONIC DISEASES

- Our vital force cannot overcome even the slightest diseases (Acute/ Chronic) & restore some sort of health without sacrificing a part of the organism (system/solid/fluid) through crisis.
- The organism usually sacrifices the least important organ/system & saves the vital system/organs.
- That is why the first manifestation of any chronic disease is on skin/mucous membranes which may be called as

EXTERIORISATION. [It can also be ELIMINATION in the form of various discharges]

	THE PLANES HUMAN EXISTENCE	Disorder First at Vital Plane	Exteriorisation
Layer 4	THE PLANE OF MIND		
Layer 2	THE PLANE OF DYNAMIS/VITAL FORCE		
Layer 3 Central Controlling axis	CNS		
	ANS		
	ENDOCRINE		
Layer 1 The Body Matrix	HUMORAL		
	VISCERAL		
	MECHANICAL		
	SKIN		

Figure 15: Elimination Vs Suppression

PROGRESSION OF CHRONIC DISEASE

- EXTERNAL LOCAL ERUPTION (After the miasma has tainted the whole organism)
- SUPPRESSION (Topical / Toxic Suppressive Treatment)
- APPARENT CURE/SLUMBERING PSORA/LATENT PSORA
- OUTBURST OF PSORA (Under conductive circumstance slumbering psora may outburst in manifold variations in accordance with individual constitution & peculiar disposition of the patient)
- VICARIOUS LOCAL MANIFESTATION
- VARIOUS INTERNAL PSORIC CONDITIONS

I shall now illustrate excerpts from the chapter Psora from Hahnemann's Nature of Chronic Disease.

The living organism is thus silently penetrated by the infection of Psora, and endeavours to relieve itself and silence the internal symptoms by the production of the local cutaneous eruption; and so long as this exists in its original form, the internal psora, with its secondary affections, cannot burst forth.

It takes from six to ten days to produce this external cutaneous symptom, and its appearance is ushered in by slight feverish symptoms, which the patient often does not notice, or merely thinks them the premonitory symptoms of an ordinary cold. The vesicles produced contain a lymph or purulent fluid, which is the infecting agent. As long as the original eruption continues the diseases is communicable by infection, but if this has disappeared, the secondary psoric symptoms, like the secondary syphilitic, are no longer capable of propagating the disease.

Whilst the primary eruption continues, the disease is most readily cured by means of the specific medicines. If no remedies be employed, then the disease increases in extent both internally and externally. The external disease increases pari passu with the internal, and silences the letter and keeps it in the latent form. All this time the individual is apparently in good health, with the exception of his external eruption of itch, the intense and intolerable itching of which at length drive him to seek medical aid.

The sole treatment of medical practitioners consists in driving the eruption off the skin as quickly as possible, which is easily affected by means of ointments or lotions; the skin is cleared, but the internal psoric disease, having now no vicarious external malady, has full leave to develop itself in the interior, and this internal psora is the essence the many thousand forms of chronic non-venereal disease.

The suppression of the itch-disease, while still recent and of very small extent, is not attended with such immediate bad effects as that of a very copious eruption of long continuance, still the danger is only more remote, not less great, for the small amount of psoric internal disease goes on silently by unmistakable signs, and if not specifically cured lasts until the very end of life.

Still the internal psoric disease, even while latent, betrays its existence by many unequivocal symptoms, though not constituting any formal disease. In different individuals these symptoms of the latent diseases are different.

WHAT HAPPENS WHEN SKIN DISEASE IS SUPPRESSED?[13]

It is remarkable how extremes meet in Hahnemann's mental organisation. In his homoeopathic law of Similia we have the principle of extreme, we might say excessive, individualization, whilst the psora-theory is an illustration of the opposite extreme of generalization.

Hahnemann had before this in his coffee-theory of chronic diseases, which he afterwards retracted in favour of psora, exhibited the same tendency to generalize, and the incubation period of his coffee-theory, curiously enough, corresponds, almost precisely with that of his psora-theory.

Thus he tells us that psora theory occupied his thoughts for about twelve years before he gave it to world, and we have evidence from his writings that the coffee-theory engaged his attention for a nearly equal period. Thus we find in his *Friend of health*, published in 1792, various hints as to coffee being at the root of many chronic diseases, and his famous essay on the manifold hurtful effects of this common beverage was published in 1803; and we have seen that the germ of his psora-theory, which was finally promulgated in 1828, is discoverable in an essay he wrote in 1816. It would had been a great boon to pathological science had Hahnemann, in place of confounding all skin diseases, and endeavored to discover the particular internal diseases with which it is possible each is in a certain measure connected.

I was glad to observe, that a beginning in this direction was made by Dr. Nunez of Madrid. He therein endeavored to show the connection of herpetic and other eruption with internal diseases, according to the portion of body they occupied. The following is a summary of Dr. Nunez's observation with reference to the connection between the seat of cutaneous affection and the internal organ affected. Of course they will require confirmation by other observers before they can be received and undoubted facts.

1. When herpetic eruptions, especially eczema on the anus and scrotum, are driven off, there follow, sooner or later, serious, even organic, liver diseases. On the other hand, liver complaints are often materially benefited by the appearance of herpes on the anus.

2. The suppression of herpes on the lower extremities, especially the legs, is often followed by liver complaints, but more frequently by affections of the stomach and other parts of the digestive organs (the bowels).

3. Prurigo on the scrotum and penis has a relation to impotence and seminal emissions. The former he found always to depend on such herpetic eruptions, when debauchery was not the cause of it.

4. The disappearance of eczema behind the ears in children is frequently by troublesome cough.

5. Phthisis pulmonalis is a frequent consequence of suppressed eruptions on the head, especially tinea.

6. The suppression of humid herpetic eruption on the arms and hands disposes the phthisis laryngea, and, on the other hand, affections of the larynx are often relieved by the appearance of eruptions on the arm.

7. The suppression of dry eruptions (lichen) on the palm of the hand often causes nervous asthma.

8. Eye affections of children and scrofulous subjects are often connected with eruptions behind the ears.

9. Seats in the nose and nostrils and erysipelatous swellings of the nose have a connection with discharges from the ears.

10. Acne rosacea and certain heart affections have a mutual dependency.

This is subject well worthy the attention of practitioners and careful may yet be productive of useful practical results, for it cannot be doubted that many chronic maladies are connected with cutaneous affections of different sorts, just as many acute febrile disease have their peculiar exanthemata.

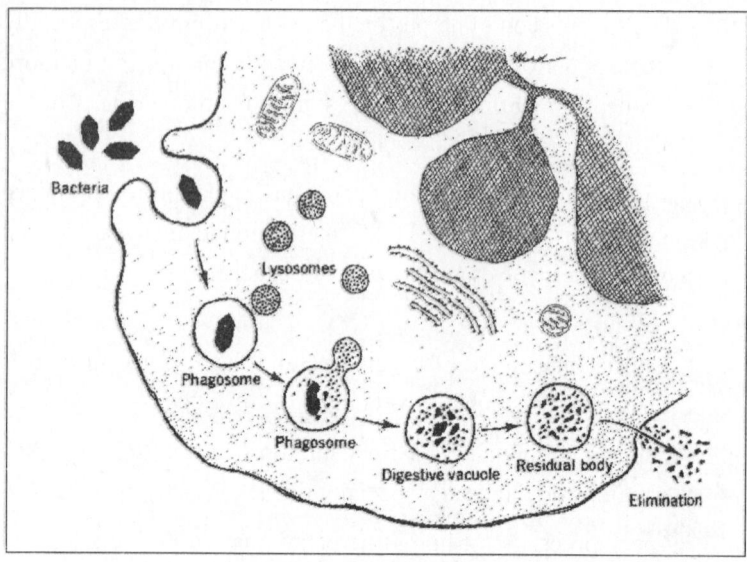

Figure 16: Elimination at cellular level

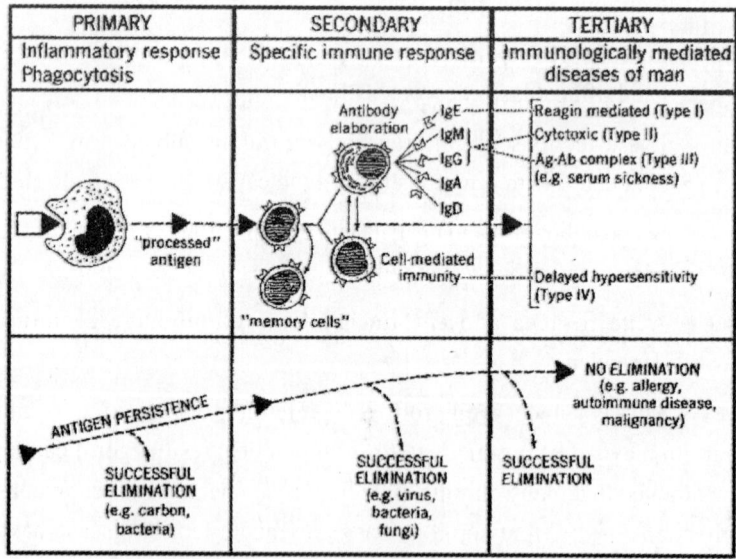

Figure 17: Elimination at immunological level

SUPPRESSION AT IMMUNOLOGICAL LEVEL

The basic function of immune system is successful elimination of all foreign (non-self) material. As it is clear from the figure 16 & 17 if there is faulty elimination or their is suppression this leads to a host of diseases like allergy, auto immune disease, malignancy.

Now what are sites of immunological elimination? Four organ-system are important, the renal-excretory mechanism, the gastro intestinal-excretory mechanism, the respiratory system and the whole of skin and of course various discharges like vaginal discharge. So finally we have immunological basis of the Homoeopathic theory of suppression. The only thing to remember is that our theory encompasses not only immunological suppression, suppression of physiological discharges (like; menses or perspiration). Pathological discharges (like leucorrhoea) but goes one step ahead and talk of suppression of mental phenomenon like suppressed grief or mortification, which psycho neuro immunology is exploring & and in just finding a link between genesis of chronic disease with psychological suppression.

Chapter 31

The Eizayaga Model of Layers of Disease[18,25]

Whilst several notable practitioner have acknowledge the existence of "Layered" cases, we are indebted to Dr. Eizayaga of Argentina for creating it. Dr. Eizayaga has clarified the different levels of activity that a miasms may manifest. There are four main categories of layer to be considered. 1. Lesion layer 2. Fundamental layer 3. Constitutional layer 4. Miasmatic layer. Each of the these terms has distinct meaning when used in the context of model and it is important not to confuse these meanings with other interpretations of the same words.

Below are the key components of each of the four major layers. The prescribing rules are different depending on which layer is being treated, so these are include under each heading.

1. LESION LAYER

When a disease process has localized in a system, apparatus, organ or tissue, it is known as a lesion and may have to be treated separately from the other layers.

A lesion may be either acute (e.g. appendicitis) or chronic (e.g. arthritis) It may be further categorized as sporadic (appearing at unpredictable intervals e.g. gout); periodic appearing at regular interval or under predictable circumstances (e.g. asthma) or permanent (e.g. cancer).

The lesion layer prescription is base upon the clinical diagnosis, the symptoms of the disease and all local modalities, concomitants and alterations. Thus the hierarchy of symptoms is the reverse of that use in constitutional prescribing. Only those mental and general symptoms are utilized, which have appeared or become worse since the disease existed.

The purpose of the treatment is to remove the disease before curing the patient. Any remedy in the Materia Medica may be used, including organ remedies and those minor remedies having clinical indications only.

In some cases sub-lesions are added to the picture and may require treatment before the lesion layer itself can be tackled. For example diabetes may be the lesion to be treated, but there are now added ulcers or visual impairment as a result of the diabetes. Similarly, a patient with cancer as the lesion layer may have just completed a course of chemotherapy or radiation, which can add a sub-lesion to the picture.

The basic rule in lesional cases is always to start with the most recent and /or most limiting problem and to work back from there. The guidelines for lesion layer prescribing are virtually identical to those that apply to the fundamental layer.

As the vast majority of chronic lesional cases will have been subject to drugs and other treatments, the repeated-low-potency approach is extremely useful from the point of view of case management.

2. FUNDAMENTAL LAYER

This layer refers mostly to functional symptoms on a mental, emotional or physical level. These are acquired characteristics and can change throughout a person's life. Symptoms on this level are relate to the person rather than to any disease process, but they are deviations from that persons's healthy state.

This layer tends to overlap with the Kentian 'constitutional' picture, and the standard Kentian hierarchy of symptoms is usually applied. Commonly this layer is found to have resulted from an emotionally etiology such as grief, anger, fright etc. food cravings and intolerances belong here, as these are not considered to be compatible with good heath. All symptoms of this layer are generally reversible and curable.

The purpose of the treatment is to remove functional disorders and to restore the patient to their original constitutional picture. Approximately thirty to forty polycrest remedies are most commonly used whose psychological picture are well-defined, such as *Pulsatilla, Natrium Mur., Stramonium, Aurum, Lachesis* etc..

3. CONSTITUTIONAL LAYER

This layer refer to what are basically healthy characteristics, and mostly they are genetic and immovable. These include the body type, hair colour basic character/personality type, food desires and aversions, and general modalities such as related to temperature and climate. All signs and symptoms on this level are compatible with good health that is why they are neither pathological not curable.

The purpose of treatment on this layer is preventive, i.e. to strengthen and fortify the constitution and thereby helping the person to keep healthy. Only a few basic polycrest remedies are used. As might be expected, babies and children are very commonly treated on the level, whereas most adults have acquired other layers, which have to be removed before the underlying constitution can be treated.

Generally speaking, one or a few doses of the indicated remedy are given in a potency from the 30th upwards the remedy may be repeated periodically in the same or a higher potency provided the person remains in good health.

4. MIASMATIC LAYER

Five basic miasmatic or 'soil' types are recognized, each producing as predisposition to certain type of disease. The general indications for each are given below:

Psora: Skin problems, itch, seasonal allergies, digestive problems, assimilation and elimination.

Sycosis: Disorder of genitals, joints and mucous membrane, benign tumors, warts, catarrhal states and obsession.

Syphilis: Self-destructive tendencies, suicide, accidents, ulcerations, necrosis and suppuration.

Tuberculosis: Respiratory problems, nasal, bronchial, pulmonary and allergies.

Cancer: Morbidity, obsessiveness, suppressions, moles and pre-cancerous states.

The majority of people deemed to have more than one miasm, and the rule of thumbs is to treat the most active or uppermost first, as and when it is encountered. However, Eizayaga suggests that it is also a good policy to treat miasmatically after the patient is fully cured, in order to consolidate the cure and reduce the likelihood of a relapse. There are three basic level of activity that may apply to a miasm:

DORMANT MIASM

This means that the miasm is indicated by the family history of the patient, or by the previous illnesses suffered by the patient, but there is no evidence that the miasm is active at the present time. The best approach with dormant miasms is to let sleeping dogs lie. If a dormant miasm is treated with the related nosode it may be activated and while this could be argued to be in the long-term interest of the patient, they are unlikely to see it that way.

ACTIVE MIASM

This means that the miasm is actively (i.e. currently) producing a tendency to certain problems, which continue to recur inspite of homoeopathic treatment.

An active miasm may also prevent will-indicated remedies from acting curatively or may provoke frequent and early relapse. This type of miasm should be treated with one or few doses of the appropriate nosode in a potency from the 30th upwards. This is usually done intercurrently during treatment of another layer and that treatment should be resumed, giving the same potency as had previously acted, shortly after the nosode had been given.

The purpose of the intercurrent miasmatic treatment is to reduce the activity of the miasm so that indicated remedies may be given with grater benefit.

EXPOSED MIASM

When a miasm is exposed, this means that the picture presenting is of the corresponding nosode- that is to say, the patient is presenting a clear picture of, say *Medorrhinum* or T*uberculinum*, with the mental state, food desire and other characteristic symptoms of the remedy. This is the only time in this model when a major nosode would be given as a first remedy and Eizayaga recommends it to be given in these case using the ascending potency scale as described above.

Chapter 32

How to Recognize Miasma by Symptomatology[1,5,11,14,15,22,23,26,27,31,32,35,38,43,47,49]

Hahnemann recognized a miasm as a disorderly state of the whole living organism, to which he ascribes the disease conditions which supervene.

These conditions, being confined within certain limits, can be classified under the three headings of psora, sycosis, and syphilis, each of which has its own stamp or individuality.

In Hahnemann's description of symptoms, the psoric so far outnumber the sycotic and the syphilitic. This, indeed, was Hahnemann's view, as he ascribed seven-eighths of chronic disease to psora and the remaining eighth to sycosis and syphilis combined.

However, on examination of the symptoms given by Hahnemann under the heading of psora we should be inclined to include some of them rather under sycosis and syphilis.

Let us now try to outline a picture of each of these chronic miasms, in order that by comparing them with the drug pictures given in our material medica we may demonstrate how the characteristics of the miasm reappear in the similimum.

SYMPTOMS OF PSORIC MIASM

SKIN

1. The skin is itchy, hot and burning, either with or without eruptions.
2. Itching is relieved by scratching, followed by burning and smarting. Worse in the evening, especially in heat of bed.
3. Dry, rough appearance of the skin dirty look, worse by washing.
4. Papular eruption present with scales and crusts are thin and fine, never thick and heavy.

FACE

1. The face may be pale, but the lips, like other mucous membranes, are very red.

EAR NOSE EYES

1. Special sense organs are not typically affected in psora.
2. Congestive conditions may lead to epistaxis and noises in the ears.
3. Itching heat, with dryness and redness, may occur on the eyelids and in the auditory meatus.

MOUTH

1. A burnt taste is the only characteristic one.

HEAD

1. Hair is dry, lusterless and brittle, with seldom any sweating of the head.

2. Frequently there is much itching of the scalp.
3. Little desire for heat about the head, the patient preferring to have the head uncovered.
4. Headaches on waking in the morning; they increase towards noon, when they reach their height then decrease towards evening. Congestive type, usually frontal or temporal. Frequently they are periodic and occur once per week or once per month, with bilious attacks, nausea and vomiting. The pain is generally relieved by hot applications, quiet, rest, and sleep.

GENERALS

1. Hot flushes are particularly common.
2. Often there is constant chilliness in these cases, but little or no sweating, which, if it occurs at all, relieves the patient.

MENTAL & SENSORIUM

1. Mentally these patients are active, self-centred, hypochondriac, changeable and moody.
2. Commonly they are morose, lazy and apathetic. They are sensitive to outside impressions, such as noises and odours, and faint easily with excitement.
3. With the moodiness and depression they may be subject to hysteria, fits of passion, tremble and weep.
4. Chronic complainers who feel they will never get well. Vertigo is common and occurs at all times and in all circumstances, accompanied or not by nausea.
5. Vertigo and nausea in boat, train, or carriage is characteristic.

G.I.T

1. Appetite may be absent or ravenous, and occur at unusual times, frequently between meals or at night.
2. Appetite may be small while thirst is great.
3. Craving for sweets is a typical psoric symptom.
4. Rich, much seasoned, and fried foods are greatly desired, and frequently lead to bilious attacks or diarrhoea.
5. Bloating and drowsiness after meals is typical of psora.
6. Diarrhoea may also follow fright or grief, and is accompanied by colicky pains which are better from hot drinks or hot applications.
7. Constipation is frequent, the desire for stool being absent, and the motion hard dry balls, as if burnt.
8. Itching, creeping, and crawling in the rectum may be present, either with or without worms

GENITALIA

1. Dysmenorrhoea may occur, but is not characteristic of psora;
2. Clots are usually small and leucorrhoea bland.

RESPIRATORY

1. Affections are of congestive type
2. Cough dry, teasing, spasmodic, with little expectoration, worse in the morning.

EXTREMITIES

1. The hands and feet are often cold, In spite of the coldness of the hands and feet, they may become extremely hot, dry, and

burning, especially in the palms and soles. This is most marked at night, and may force the patient to put the feet from under the covers to cool them off.
2. Tingling and numbness in the limbs, which easily become weary, especially with standing; the patient can walk well cannot stand well.
3. Chillblains are common, and burn and itch.
4. Disagreeable odour from the feet.
5. Limb pains, like the headache, are better from heat, rest, and quiet; and worse from motion.

SYMPTOMS OF SYCOTIC MIASM

1. Sycosis has been defined as the fig-wart disease.
2. The signature of the disease is still the warty growths.

SKIN

1. The skin is oily, greasy, and sallow, or of a peculiar waxy greenish hue.
2. In extreme cases a general puffiness or doughiness may be found.
3. Blemishes on the skin are frequent, and may appear as little red polka dots or sycotic moles, spider spots, naevi, or brown patches.
4. Red moles are frequent on neck, chest, and trunk.
5. In sycosis, vesicular eruptions are characteristic, and may become pustular, as in herpes, impetigo, and vaccinia. Itching is usually absent in these cases
6. Warts of all kinds and in all situations ate typically sycotic. They may be pigmented, disseminated, unilateral or in groups.

7. *Tinea barbae* and *Tinea circumscripta*, the latter leading to bald spots on the scalp, are due to this miasm only.

8. Nails are usually thick and ridged.

GENERALS

1. Perspiration is frequently profuse, both day and night, on scalp, trunk, and genitals. The odour may be musty or fishy. The perspiration does not relieve the patient.

2. These patients are usually chilly and sensitive to cold and damp, but despite this fact, children frequently kick off all the covers at night.

3. There is constantly are always worse before change of weather, or approach of thunderstorm, and are noticeably present with the pains.

4. One of the chief differences between psora and sycosis is here exemplified. Psora seldom produces pathological states, being more functional in its effects, while sycosis is rapid in action and produces pathological results more rapidly even than syphilis.

MENTALS

1. The mental states of sycosis are related chiefly to meninges, hence convulsions and epileptiform seizures are common.

2. The patient is nervous, excitable, irritable, emotional, and easily startled by noises.

HEAD

1. Headaches are frontal, occipital or on vertex, and are worse from barometric changes and moisture of atmosphere. Heat does not always relieve the pain; motion frequently does.

EYES

1. Ophthalmia with profuse purulent greenish discharge may occur;
2. Also corneal ulcer and iritis.

EARS

1. Otitis media of a chronic type with purulent discharge is often of sycotic origin.

NOSE

1. The nose shares in the general catarrhal state of the miasm, acute or chronic catarrh being practically constant.
2. Acute coryza with sneezing and copious watery excoriating discharge is followed by, or replaced by, stuffy catarrh after the least exposure to cold.

DIGESTIVE

1. Appetite is usually capricious, and frequently entirely absent in the morning.
2. Indigestion after food is a frequent complaint.
3. Fruit in particular seems to upset some of these patients.
4. With infants, even the mother's milk may upset, and one finds a new-born infant screaming and squirming, with the legs drawn up on the abdomen. This continues for hours unless relived. Milk foods in general disagree with these infants, consequently feeding is very difficult. The stomach pains are crampy, colicky, Paroxysmal, and are relived by pressure, lying on the abdomen, motion, or rocking. Vomiting may occur, and both the child and the vomitus smell sour. The child does not want to be left alone, but wants to be carried or rocked.

5. Diarrhea is one of the outstanding features of sycosis, and may follow trivial causes such as any indiscretion in diet or a wetting.
6. The stool is forcibly ejected with much pain and noise; smells sour, and is acid and corrosive. The colour and consistency are not characteristic, and may be watery, white, green, or yellow.
7. The type of colic is extremely severe, spasmodic, paroxysmal, and is relieved by hard pressure, such as bending over the back of a chair, and is accompanied by much restlessness.
8. J. H. Allen says appendicitis is largely dependent on the sycotic miasm.
9. Stitching pains, especially in rectum and vagina, may occur.
10. Pruritus ani and vulvae when present are very severe.
11. Umbilicus and rectum may be the site of ulceration with a thin watery discharge.
12. When Haemorrhoids are present, they are characterized by intense pruritus.

KIDNEY

1. Kidney involvement may be found in markedly sycotic cases, leading to dropsy, etc.
2. The urine, like the stool, is so acrid that great care is necessary to prevent excoriation about the perineum.
3. Pain on passing urine may be so extreme as to cause children to scream.

GENITALIA

1. Sycosis characteristically affects the whole pelvic cavity leading to any or all of the following conditions: metritis, para and endo-metritis, salpingitis, ovaritis, etc.

2. This leads to extreme dysmenorrhea with the type of pain already detailed under colic.
3. The flow may occur only with the pains, and is usually offensive, acrid, and excoriating. Typically, it contains large, dark, stringy clots.
4. Leucorrhea is also acrid, thin, scanty, and of a typical fishy odour.

EXTREMITIES

1. The extremities exemplify the tendency of the miasm to affect fibrous tissue.
2. Shooting and tearing pains occur in the muscles and joints of the extremities, accompanied by stiffness and soreness, especially lameness.
3. Small joints are frequently selected, such as the finger joints, the forefinger being a common seat of election.
4. The soles of the feet are painful and tender, and the patient may complain of the sensation of walking on cobbles.
5. These pains are worse from rest as the affected parts stiffen up, so that while the pains are relieved by motion, they are very much aggravated on beginning to move.
6. These pains, like most other sycotic conditions, are worse from cold, barometric changes, especially damp, and better in dry fair weather and from motion. They may be worse at night or in the morning.
7. The general restlessness of the miasm is seen particularly in the feet, and may even be exaggerated to choreiform movements.
8. Chronic joint inflammation is never grossly deforming, as it attacks the fibrous tissues in and around the joints. In pursuance of this tendency to affect fibrous tissue, nerve sheaths and muscle tendons may be affected.

9. In acute articular rheumatism the joints are swollen, blue and sensitive, and the inflammation may move from joint to joint.
10. In sycosis, in contrast to the tubercular diathesis, there is an increase in the amount of chalk deposited which leads to nodules round joints and in muscle sheaths.

RESPIRATORY SYSTEM

1. The respiratory tract is much involved in the general catarrhal state of mucous membranes, which show a typical patchy bluish congestion. The whole tract is frequently involved, nasal catarrh being followed by bronchitis, accompanied by a hard, dry, racking cough. Asthma is a purely sycotic manifestation, especially the humid type which is hereditary. There is prolonged teasing cough with little expectoration, which may be clear mucus or ropy. Time aggravation of asthma and cough is frequently 2 to 3 a.m. Endocardium and pericardium may be involved and lead to sudden death, with no pain and few symptoms. Pain may be present in the scapular and precordial regions. There is one other disease which is capable of attacking all these tissues susceptible to attack under sycosis, and that disease is influenza, which is one of the outstanding sycotic affections.

SYMPTOMS OF SYPHILITIC MIASM

SKIN

1. The skin lesions in syphilis are polymorphic, copper or raw-ham coloured, symmetrical, and devoid of pain or itching.
2. Scales and crusts, when present, tend to be thick and heavy, as in rupia. Pearly papules and leucoplachia carry the stamp of the miasm.

3. Onychia, paronychia, and dactylitis also tell their own tale.

FACE

1. The face is ashy grey, wizened and wrinkled, giving in children the typical "old man" appearance.

MENTALS

1. The syphilitic miasm leads to a dull, heavy mentality.
2. The sufferer is sullen and obstinate.
3. He is mistrustful.
4. Depression may be so intense as to lead to suicide.
5. Anxiety at night is so marked that the syphilitic dreads the night.

HEAD

1. Headaches are basilar, dull, constant, and may persist for days. The pain becomes worse towards evening; increases till midnight, and eases off towards morning. Lying down and heat both aggravate, while cold usually alleviates the pain.
2. The pain may be so severe that a child knocks its head against the sides of the cot or with its hands.
3. The head is large and bossy (soft) with an oily scalp, which may have thick, moist, heavy yellow crusts on it.

EYES

1. In the eyes we find many characters of the miasm, keratitis being the typical affection, which usually occurs between the ages of 7 and 21 years.

2. Iritis also is of frequent occurrence, as at least 50 percent. Of these cases of these condition have behind them the syphilitic miasm. An infant aged 6 to 9 months may show signs of iritis.

3. Syphilitic iritis is usually bilateral. The pain is like other syphilitic pains, worse at night, especially between 2 a.m. 5 a.m.

4. Ulceration of the cornea may occur with marked photophobia, but is not so common as in the tuberculous diathesis.

5. Ptosis and ciliary neuralgias are frequent manifestations.

NOSE

1. The bones of the nose are often destroyed, which results in the typical sunken bridge in children.

2. Eyebrows and eyelashes may fall out.

3. In adults, the sense of smell may be lost.

4. Nasal catarrh is frequent; acute with discharge which fluent, acrid discharge or chronic catarrh with discharge which is dark, thick and leads to the formation of clinkers.

5. The discharge is not always offensive.

MOUTH

1. Moist ulceration and mucous patches are common on tongue, gums, palate and tonsils, giving the characteristic snail-track appearance.

2. Dentition is troublesome; diarrhoea and convulsions being frequent accompaniments.

3. Hutchinson's peg teeth are known to all.

4. A metallic taste in the mouth always suggests syphilis.

5. Enlargement of the cervical glands, most often those in the posterior triangle and behind the ear.

ALIMENTARY SYSTEM

1. The digestive and Alimentary systems are not characteristically affected, but marasmic children may develop sudden attacks of severe vomiting and purging which may be fatal in twenty- four hours unless checked.

EXTREMITIES

1. Both upper and lower, are typical sites of bone pains, which may or may not be accompanied by thickening and deformity.
2. Ulceration of the long bones frequently follows, ulcer in the upper third of the tibia being diagnostic.
3. The bone pains are like the head pains-worse at night, and ameliorated by cold.

RESPIRATORY SYSTEM

1. Laryngeal affections are the chief of the manifestations of the miasm in the respiratory system, and may be functional or destructive.

SYMPTOMS OF TUBERCULAR MIASM

This brief survey of the miasm of syphilis brings to mind the miasm of tubercle which is in many ways very similar.

This fact is acknowledged by all schools of medicine, sometimes the difficulty of distinguishing their products being extreme.

J.H. Allen in his book on "Psora and Pseudo-Psora" ascribes to a mixture of psora and syphilis with the miasm scrofula, and Osler has said that scrofula is tubercle.

Is it surprising then that the miasm of tubercle contains symptoms of more than one miasm, and that it is of deadly significance, always predisposing to extremes? This is seen particularly in the acute exanthemata, where the attack is always severe, and tends to be followed by secondary complications.

It is not included by Hahnemann in his triad of chronic basic miasms, but its presence is so widespread that it may not be out of place to include it here as one of the basic constitutional derangements.

Here, however, one may add that no claim is made that these miasms dealt with complete the list of chronic miasms, but it is hoped that sufficient evidence has been put forward to show that their presence is no mean factor in the diseases and disorders with we have daily to deal.

Let us now proceed to outline the miasm of tubercle.

SKIN

1. Skin lesions are multiform and generally free from itch. Ringworm, purpura, erythema nodosum, and eczema may all occur.

FACE

1. The face is typically pale with a clear, watery, bluish tint;
2. Bright eyes with long lashes, and high cheek bones which may show the typical malar flush.
3. The lips are frequently bright red, but may be congested and blue.

GENERALS

1. The patient is either too fat or too thin, too dull or too active, and always too tired.

2. Muscle and fat predominate, tissues are lax, and bones soft and rickety.
3. These patients constantly chilly, susceptible to the least cold, yet upset by extreme heat.
4. Perspiration is free about the face, head, and upper part of the body. The odour may be offensive, especially that of the feet.
5. Feet and hands are cold and clammy
6. Lymphatic tissue is typically affected all over the body-tonsils and adenoids, cervical glands, mesenteric glands, all become enlarged.

MENTALS

1. The mental symptoms are pronounced in children who are often willful, stubborn, positive, and bad tempered, and may also be destructive. They may be weepy and full of fears and dreads; fear of animals being marked. At night want to be carried, as in sycosis; they prefer not to be touched.
2. Older patients may be hopeful in outlook, even with marked constitutional disturbance.
3. Hysteria may occur, and is generally a danger signal.
4. Epilepsy may develop at, or about, puberty.

HEAD

1. Tubercular Headaches are very severe, frequently periodic, or are brought on by an excitement or strain. Heat, rest and quiet ameliorate the pains, as does eating. They are usually frontal or temporal.

NOSE

1. Catarrhal affections of the nose frequently occur, either acute or chronic, the latter with thick yellow discharge, which may smell of old cheese.

EYE

1. The most characteristic condition is phlyctenular ulcer with intense photophobia.

EAR

1. Affections are common after the slightest exposure to cold, and the child wakes up screaming during the night. The discharge, here as elsewhere, may smell like old cheese.
2. Cracks behind the ears frequently occur.

DIGESTIVE SYSTEM

1. Ravenous appetite, especially for indigestible things, such as chalk, pencils, and craving for meat is common.
2. Salt is much desired and much needed.
3. Sudden attacks of vomiting and diarrhoea may follow any chill, error in diet, and teething.
4. Stools may be clay-coloured, and contain blood and mucus.
5. Intestinal parasites are of common occurrence.

KIDNEY

1. Bladder and kidney involvement frequently leads to enuresis.
2. Diabetes frequently has a tubercular basis.

GENITAL SYSTEM

1. Menses are exhausting, frequent, profuse, and may be accompanied by nausea, fainting or hysterical symptoms.
2. Leucorrhoea is usually thick, musty, purulent and lumpy.

EXTREMITIES

1. In the limbs, owing to the laxity of the tissues, sprains and strains are common, also, the patient may stumble over a straw.
2. Bony tissues are markedly affected, the spine and long bones, especially near joints, being the seats of affection.
3. There is deficiency in chalk and silicates, and nails are brittle, frequently with white spots or excessive curves, concave or with clubbing of the finger ends.

SYMPTOMS OF CANCER MIASM

[Comments From: Dr. Mortelmans Guido – (MG)/Dr. Smits Tinus- (ST)/Dr. Degroote Filip- (DF)/Dr. Peters Rob- (PR)/Dr. Geukens Alfons- (GA)/Dr. Kokelenberg Guy- (KG)/Dr. Gaublomme Kris- (GK) Dr. de Bacts Piet- (DBP)/Dr. Scheepers Leon – (SL)/Dr. van Hootegen Henk- (VHN)/Dr. Foubister- (FB)]

MIND

1. *Anxiety:* People having anxiety about their family, about others, because the family protects him.
2. *Clairvoyance:* During their life and it has something to do with the anxiety, some strange talents, gifts may come out, for Example, 'Clairvoyance'. At a Certain moment of their life they will have Clairvoyance. Mostly, They will have Clairvoyance in Their dream, not Knowing about it, because they Wake in the morning and When you ask them about their dream, They won't know it. – (KG)
3. *Not easily Satisfied:* one of the things that strike is the fact that they are not easily satisfied. They are rather Critical Persons. They like to make little remarks, and Corrections, like an old-School teacher. – (KG)

4. *Fear of Failure:* He has the Fear of failure of *Lycopodium*. He had the delusion he will never reach his destination. He wants to be perfect and cannot be so.

5. *Domination:* excessive parental Control; long history of domination: When there is too much control of the environment on the child it can suffer and bring out the disease.

6. *Fastidious:* the Fastidiousness in cancer miasm is very Characteristic. They can be very fastidious in their work, what they make. But they can rather be untidy in their house, not arrange their affairs. But if it Concerns something that expresses their Personality, it must be perfect. It is not like *Arsenicum*. They must have all the things in their Place. The *Carcinosin* patient is doing something it must be perfect, while he has a great lack of confidence. If he makes something, it must be Good, so that there is no reproach to make. I can't say that *Carcinosin*- People are always well dressed. There is not that kind of fastidiousness like in *Arsenicum*. – (ST)

7. *Fear:* apprehension, dread animals, of busy streets, of Crowd, in a Dark, of dogs, of examination, before examination, of failure, of health of loved persons, about narrow Places, in Vaults, Churches and cellars for a long time, Fear of Spiders: you have to think of *Carcinosin* In Children who have nightmares. They wake up and they are afraid of Something. They think there is something in the Corner of the Room. – (FB)

8. *Horrible things; affect her profoundly:* the Symptom "horrible things affect her profoundly" is typical Cancer miasm. But I Think it is more the sensitiveness they have. Like here, she is very Sensitive to romantic films and there is feeling in it. It Must not always be horrible things. I think they are sensitive to things in general. – (MG)

9. *Irritability: morning; after rising; because of forgetfulness:* they are irritated by trifles, for example, when they go to

Sleep. They will be Disturbed by little things, by little noises far away, Some light, wrinkled bed Cloths and so on. These things disturb a Person with cancer miasm and Make him Sleepless. – (KG)

10. *Memory:* Weakness Of, for everyday things: They are Forgetful. They will forget little things, not important things. When they go Shopping they will forget little things. Or in Household affairs they will forget little things and they will be very angry about it. Angry at themselves, because they have forgotten to do Something. – (KG)

11. *Obstinate:* People with cancer miasm are known as Sensitive People, Sensitive Children, but at the same time they can be very obstinate. – (MG)

12. *Precocity:* when the patient feels very well, there is a Clairvoyance or Precocity of Mind – (DF). My opinion about one of the aspects of Precocity of people with cancer miasm is that they begin to Masturbate very Soon, Their Sexuality Is very early developed in life. It is Responsibility that makes them grown up sooner. It is as if the hormones Starts Sooner – (KG). He is Precocious on the Sexual Sphere. He Starts to masturbate very early. Very young Children, even if they are only 2 yrs. Old, he is very Precocious in reading. (Paschero & Cahiers Hahnemannians of Lyon)

13. *Passion to read:* another Symptom for people with cancer miasm is a passion to read. A Lot of Children read, But if a Child is reading real books, no Comic Strips or adventures, but all kinds of books, then think of *Carcinosin*. – (MG) I Suggest to Make a new addition in 'Play, indisposition to". – (DBP)

14. *Sensitive; oversensitive to Music, to Noise, to Reprimands:* don't get the False impression that they are very Serious, depressed people. No. They are Very Lively Persons, Very Sensitive Persons,They Love Music, They Love to

Sing, They Love to dance, along with a partner, They are Very Romantic, very Sentimental, Very Sensitive to Overwhelming Things. For Example, They can Stand before a Waterfall and Get chills, just by Seeing the immense Power of the waterfall or for Example, in a Airport, an aeroplane that is landing, they will watch it and will get tears in their eyes, just by Seeing it or a Parade, Olympic Games, an orchestra. They are Very Sensitive to overwhelming, important things. They get goose-flesh from it, or Chills, or They will weep, "Weeping From Music" is an addition for *Carcinosin*. They Like To watch a Lightning and a Thunderstorm. It is the Some thing. – (KG). Lightening important. *Carcinosin* People are Known as Sensitive People, Sensitive children, but at the same time they can be very Obstinate. That is also one of the things we Know of *Carcinosin*. If they are Suppressed as a Child, if they Have a dictatorial father or Mother, They can not show their feelings because they are so sensitive. – (MG)

15. *Suicidal; disposition; cancer history in the Family, with:* People who need *Carcinosin* in Their Family history There was Cancer or Leukemia, or Tuberculosis, Pernicious anaemia. It is Curious, Such a Child whose mother died from Cancer and I was Looking in my practice to find children or people who have the same appearance of the Children whose mother were Suffering from cancer during pregnancy and I gave the remedy *Carcinosin*. – (FB)

16. *Talk, indisposed to, desire to be silent:* about the depression of *Carcinosin*; They are closed up, they Won't Talk about it, they don't like any fuss about it, leave me alone, no Consolation please and "don't want to talk" I don't want to see anybody, I work it out myself. Because the depression has come, they want to overcome the influence of others, they don't want others to influence them in their depression. That's why

Carcinosin is in "consolation agg." They love people, and they are very open and Sympathetic and Sentimental, but when the depression has Come, they do not want anybody to interfere with. They are a bit like Sepia. And the depression will be very deep. It may lead to Suicide like *Aurum*. It is a very Serious problem. – (KG)

17. *Thunderstorm, loves:* Cheerful when it thunders and at Lightening. – (DBP).

18. *Tidy:* this is also a Point of *Carcinosin*. Most of the Children are not tidy but if they are very tidy, it is a Symptom. Also *Carcinosin* can have that. You can add it in the rubric "Conscientious about trifles." – (MG)

EYE

1. Blueness, Conjunctiva, Sclera: First there is appearance and facies, I already talked about. It is only very Suggestive when you see blue Sclerotics, or moles, or acne or tics, like blinking with his eyes, tapping with his fist on his head, biting nails and so on. – (DF)

FACE

1. Discolouration; bluish, lips; brown (Coffee Coloured); Café au lait Complexion and moles. – (FB)

STOMACH

1. Anxiety: Fear that is left in the Stomach, is a Symptom that is known for *Carcinosin*. He says "anxiety." The fear used as a Symptom when the fear is felt as a Constriction in the stomach region. When the Patient is telling you this, you may use the rubric, "Fear felt in Stomach." When they say, "When I am not feeling easy, and I feel Something in my

stomach." It is more anxiety felt in the stomach. That is really what Foubister said, that is really *Carcinosin*. The real fear is one second going down to the stomach is known for *Carcinosin*. – (DF)

2. Desires; Chocolate: the biggest desire of *Carcinosin* is Chocolate. They also like all kinds of Sweets. It is important. Another desire is meat and fat, fat meat, bacon. That is important, for example in children they like to eat fat bacon. You give *Tuberculinum* or *Calcarea phosphorica*, but there is also *Carcinosin*. 'Highly seasoned food" is also *Carcinosin*. That is from Paschero. But they also like salt. There are a lot of desire and aversions in *Carcinosin*.

3. Ulcers (Ulcer Pepticum); with a strong family history: a bad dyspepsia, an indigestion, gastroenteritis, peptic ulcers, disposition to ulcer is very strong in the family, diarrhoea, vomiting, it is also a good remedy for cyclical vomiting, diarrhoea in infancy or Childhood, chronic hepatitis, worms and Constipation, especially in children. – (DF)

4. Vomiting; alternating with diarrhoea periodic (Cyclical): here we see the connection between the cyclical vomiting and his mental overexertion. When his mind is working too much, he starts vomiting he can't stop anymore. Once he starts vomiting he has to go to the hospital for rehydration. – (DBP)

GENITALIA

1. Masturbation; disposition to in Children: That is Something I noticed in one Patient, you know the symptom in Children "disposition to Masturbation." *Carcinosin* is one of the big remedies with Medorrhinum. Also in this Case there was really an aversion to Sex. Her husband Couldn't Touch her. It was terrible. She was dreaming about having sex with him. It is very strange. It goes to the Subconscious and there is again

the sexual thing. My impression is that most of *Carcinosin* People are rather Sexual:, not very Strong. If the Sex is not expressed you see Masturbation, in this Person it Came in the Dreams. – (MG)

SKIN

1. Discoloration; brown (Coffee-Coloured):I was having a quick look at him during the Consultation. He had this beautiful café au lait discolouration in his neck. It gave me a kick. Then I heard about the chocolate, the soup, the desires and I became more and more Convinced that *Carcinosin* was definitely to be Considered. – (GK): she said it herself, coffee with milk. It is a typical a *Carcinosin* thing but Foubister said you do not need that symptom to give *Carcinosin*. He said that most of his patients did not have this "cafe-au-lait" moles, they don't have blue sclera and he gave *Carcinosin* with result. So you do not need this thing to give *Carcinosin*. – (MG)
2. Moles; Naevi: it was Foubister who came on the idea to have more information about *Carcinosin*, because among his patients he had some children whose mother suffered from cancer during Pregnancy. He recognized some features in those children. I will tell you which those remarkable features were. They will have blue Sclerotics, a café au lait Complexion, and numerous moles. – (DF).

GENERALITIES

1. Anaemia, pernicious (in family history).
2. Cancerous affections; cachexia, emaciation with aims, to relief.
3. Change, Symptoms, Constant Chronic of.
4. Children, affections in biting nails.

5. Constriction, Sensation of external.
6. Contradictory and alternating states.
7. Dwarfishness: The dwarfishness is also a typical symptom for *Carcinosin*. – (DF)
8. Inflammation, Hepatitis., Sinusitis., Tonsillitis: itching at eye corners, sneezing, bleeding gums, all these symptoms always came when she was going to have a Sinusitis. It always started with itching at the inside of her eyes, sneezing. Soon after that she had a sinusitis. All these symptoms, one after another came the first week after the remedy. It is beautiful. – (GK)
9. Mononucleosis infectiosa, acute. After-effects from; never well since: there can also be a Previous or acute mononucleosis infectiosa or frequent infective disease can also be a strong. – (DF)

Chapter 33

Key Characteristics of Miasma

THE MIASMA OF PSORA

DEFECT [DISBALANCE/DEFICIENCY]

1. Functional disorder.
2. Absence of structural disease.
3. Depletion resulting from acute disease, activity of other miasm, suppression of physical / emotional state.
4. Exhaustion & collapse.
5. Anxiety Neurosis.

LYMPHATIC DIATHESIS HISTORY OF

- Family History of Multiple allergies
- Past History of Suppressions of skin eruption

- Past history of Suppressions of physiological discharges

MIND

- Quick; Intelligent; Restless; Sensitive;
- Anxiety & Fears.
- Fear of death; Existential have aspect of psoric mentals is seen in mental state of *Psorinum*, i.e., Gloom; doom; depression; rejected & despairing & dependent on fate: NO WAY OUT.
- Delusion of being a martyr.

GENERALS

- WORSE: SUPPRESSIONS
- WORSE: COLD & DRY
- WORSE: WINTERS
- WORSE: THUNDERSTORM
- WORSE: WASHING
- AMELIORATED: PHYSIOLOGICAL DISCHARGE.
- BETTER: REST

FOOD

- DESIRES: Indigestible things warm food.
- AVERSION: Sweets, Fish.

PAIN: BURNING

DISCHARGES: Thin; Acrid; Bloody

ONSET: Early onset of clear sing & symptoms

THE MIASMA OF SYCOSIS

EXCESS [PROLIFERATION]

1. Warts/ Papilloma/ Condylomata.
2. Catarrh.
3. Genito Urinary Problems.
4. Asthma with bronchitis
5. Rheumatic Arthritis
6. Early age Myocardial ischemia
7. Obsessive Compulsive neurosis
8. Multiple fungal infections.

URIC ACID DIATHESIS HISTORY OF

- FAMILY HISTORY of Metabolic disorders [Gout RA, Stones, increased cholesterol, early age MI, Arteriosclerosis].
- FAMILY HISTORY of Gonorrhea.
- PAST HISTORY of Gonorrhea, Chronic PID, Multiple vaccination, Increased Protein & Carbohydrate Intake.
- PAST HISTORY of Suppressions of pathological discharges.

APPEARANCE

- Full body; Large full lips, Greasy Skin with dandruff, bushy eyebrows.
- Coarse facial appearance.
- Extreme sycosis: Down syndrome.

CHILDREN

- Waxy; Anaemic, Constitution poor digestion. Diarrhea with undigested food particles. Failure to thrive.

MIND

- Suspicious; Irritable; Jealous; Secretive; Deceitful; Vicious; Amoral; Obsessive with Rigid Need to Control
- SHAME is very striking
- Delusion: Immoral
- Duality of Mind: Good Vs Devil
- People of the night; Sensual & pleasure seeking
- Erratic behavior
- Fear: DOGS
- Delusion: Someone is behind them

GENERALS

WORSE: COLD & WET

WORSE: DAMP

BETTER NIGHT,

BETTER SEA

BETTER RUBBING

WORSE: COLD APPLICATION

\>> Pathological discharge.

˜ PAIN: Neuralgic/ Collie

DISCHARGES: Jelly; Acrid; Fishy

ONSET: Insidious & slow healing. Ailment in first few month of life.

THE MIASMA OF SYPHILIS

DESTRUCT [DISTORTION/DEFORMITY]

1. Ulceration.
2. Neurological disease.
3. Arterial disease [Valvular Heart Disease; Aneurysm etc.]
4. Congenital abnormality.
5. Psychosis
6. Any disease with is RAPID & DESTRUCTIVE.
7. OCD.

DYSCRATIC DIATHESIS HISTORY OF

- Family History of Degenerative Neurological disease
- Family History of Congenital birth defect
- Family History of Alcoholism
- Family History of Blood dyscrasia
- Family History of Increased incidence of suicide
- Past History of Syphilis
- Past History of Viral disease
- Past History of Suppressions of pathological discharge, pathological elimination

APPEARANCE

- Facial Asymmetry
- Look older
- Sharp/Deformed teeth

- Sigma of congestive Syphilis

CHILDREN

- Large head. Waxy & greasy hair with offensive smell. Hair falling. Failure to thrive & Marasmus
- Saddle nose. Peg teeth. Bone deformities. Congenital abnormalities

MIND

- Self destructive & paranoid.
- Show stupid Imbecile Or
- Depression; distortion; depersonalization; Suicidal; psychosis.
- Desire Death.
- Fear Night/ Illness.
- Fear Insanity/ Financial ruin Fear Robbers/ Germs.
- Delusions: Grandeur.

GENERALS

- WORSE: WARM WET
- WORSE: NIGHT
- WORSE: SEA
- THUNDER-STORM
- BETTER: MOUNTAINS
- BETTER: GENITAL MOTION [GENTLE]
- BETTER: COLD APPLICATION
- >> Pathological discharge.

FOOD: DESIRES: Aversion Meat.

PAIN: Come & go/in Straight line, Bone; lightening, deep boring pain. Sharp Stabbing, Deep Boring.

DISCHARGES: Offensive; Excoriating

ONSET: Sudden with few prodromal sign & symptoms, Congenital defect.

THE TUBERCULAR MIASM

CHANGEABLE [BURNING UP]

1. Tuberculoma.
2. Tendency to take cold.
3. Lower Respiratory Tract Infections; recurrent.
4. Lymphadenopathy.
5. Disturbed Calcium Metabolism.
6. Allergies
7. Organic endocrine disease.
8. Thyrotoxicosis
9. Organic bone disease
10. Midline congenital Abnormality.

TUBERCULAR DIATHESIS HISTORY OF

- Family History of Tuberculosis.
- Family History of Midline congenital abnormality.
- Family History of Allergies.

APPEARANCE

- Thin, emaciated, tall, stoop shouldered
- Big eyes, long eye lashes; blue sclera, red lips with white line around lips.
- Delicate white, marble like skin with tans easily.

CHILDREN

- Beautiful child as above with good teeth & chest, deformity / Midline congenital, deformity/ stoop shouldered.

MIND

- Discontented & Restless
- Obstinate changeable mood [changes jobs; friends, address, partners]
- Easily offended Fear cats [Love; Fear; Allergy]
- Fear existential
- Fear being left alone
- Delusion: Are precocious.

GENERALS

- WORSE: CHANGE OF WEATHER
- WORSE: ON WALKING
- BETTER: OPEN AIR
- BETTER: MOUNTAINS
- BETTER: FAST MOTION
- WORSE: COLD WASHING.

FOOD

- DESIRES: Ice cream, Cold Milk, Smoked Meat.
- Appetite increased yet thin.

THE CANCER MIASM

DEFENCELESS

1. Hypoglycemia.
2. Adrenal insufficiency.
3. Endometriosis + Pre Menstrual Tension.
4. Asthma [when everything fails]
5. Worms [when everything fails]
6. Scars [when everything fails]
7. Recurrent tonsils [when everything fails]
8. Chronic constipation [when everything fails]
9. Tick & Twitches.
10. Chronic Fatigue Syndrome.
11. CANCERS

CANCEROUS DIATHESIS HISTORY OF

Family History of Cancer.

Family History of Diabetes Mellitus/Tuberculosis.

Family History of Pernicious Anemia.

Family History of Rheumatic/Rheumatoid Arthritis.

Family History of Multiple allergies.

Past History of Glandular fever.

Past History of Vaccination.

Past History of Head injury.

APPEARANCE

- Intense engagement of life discontent.
- Low self esteem.
- Worried look.

CHARACTERISED BY

1. Blue Sclera.
2. Café 'au' lait spots.
3. Moles & warts.

MIND

- Intense engagement of life with discontent & low self esteem & loss of individuality.
- Sensitive to reprimands Empathy & love for others [animals] fastidious at work untidy at home, precocious, contradictory & alternating states. Many fears & conflict of loyalty.

GENERALS

WORSE/ BETTER EVENING

WORSE/ BETTER SEASIDE, SEA AIR

WORSE/ BETTER THUNDER-STORM

FOOD: WORSE/ BETTER: CHOCOLATE /SWEETS

SECTION VI: MIASMATIC CASE MANAGEMENT

Chapter 34

Hahnemannian Model of Anti-Miasmatic Treatment

Chapter 35

P.N. Banerjee on Miasmatic Case Management

Chapter 36

Miasmatic Prescribing

Chapter 34

Hahnemannian Model of Anti-Miasmatic Treatment

IN CASE OF TRUE CHRONIC MIASMATIC DISEASE[8,9]

Identify which chronic miasm is involved in the case. Whether it is syphilis or sycosis alone or it is psora complicated with syphilis or sycosis. Whether it is psora alone or complicated by allopathic treatment (Aphorism 206).

One must differentiate between actual cause of disease (fundamental cause) and occasion of the appearance of the symptoms (exciting cause). Ascertain what treatment patient has received till date. Consider the patient's circumstances and his mode of thought and emotions. Ascertain obstacles to cure. (Aphorism 206, 207, 208 and also footnote 206)

Based on the totality of symptoms start the treatment with the most homoeopathic anti-miasmatic medicine. (Aphorism 209)

In non-venereal chronic disease, those, therefore that arise from psora, we often require, in order to effect a cure, to give several antipsoric remedies in succession, every successive one being homoeopathically chosen in consonance with the group of symptoms remaining after completion of the action of the previous remedy, which may have been employed in a single dose or in several successive doses. (Aphorism 171)

IN CASE OF ACUTE EXACERBATION IN CHRONIC DISEASE[8,9]

In case of simple chronic miasmatic disease if an acute paroxysm presents after the acute exacerbation subsides by use of an Apsoric remedy give an appropriate anti-psoric.

If it is a complex chronic miasmatic disease after giving an anti-psoric follow by whatever miasma that superimposes thereafter give anti-psoric again.

IN CASE OF COMPLEX CHRONIC MIASMATIC DISEASE[8,9]

Where two dissimilar disease exists in the organism besides each other, the cure will be completely effected by a judicious alteration of the best mercurial preparation with the remedies specific for the psora, each given in the most suitable dose and form. (Foot-note Aphorism 40)

At the time when Hahnemann was practicing in Paris with his second wife Melanie (1835-43), his observation was that psora was the predominant miasm. Such was its prevalence, he felt it is necessary to treat virtually every chronic case with Sulphur, this being the major anti-psoric remedy.

His preferred method, worked out after years of experimentation, was to give Sulphur usually at the outset, either as an LM potency or a centesimal potency (up to 200) diluted in water and alcohol and repeated at regular intervals such as daily or every other day. He would continue with this until new symptoms came up or certain symptoms intensified, when he would then prescribe for the new symptoms immediately with the best indicated remedy. He would either stop the Sulphur while doing so, or in some case would continue to give it, say in LM potency continuously, while treating the new aspect of the disorder with a different remedy in a centesimal potency. Evidence suggests that Hahnemann prescribed Sulphur in this way even in cases where it did not seem at all indicted by the symptoms, so it is clear, he was prescribing on miasm-similarity rather than symptom similarity.

Chapter 35

P.N. Banerjee on Miasmatic Case Management[6]

In examining your case, you have to complete the record you have made, by ascertaining which of these miasms is or are in your patient and which of these, has the preponderance. Find out for yourself the miasmatic character of the patient from what symptoms you have already recorded.

All the three miasms have their characteristic ways of expression. The psora patient has a particular character of his diseases and symptoms, the sycotic patient has his, and the syphilitic to his. Then again, the mixed miasms-such as, Syco-psora, syphilo-psora, pseudo-psora and psora-syco-syphilis- have also their definite characters of manifestation as diseases. If you have learnt up the distinctions between the one and the other, it will not be altogether impossible for you to find out the miasmatic basis of your patient, with success.

This you have to do and add to the record you have prepared, as without knowing the miasmatic basis of the case-that is to say, without knowing that which is giving your patient a chronic disease of a particular kind, you can not make a miasmatic prescription, and unless a miasmatic prescription is made, the cure of the chronic diseases is far from hand.

If you want to trace out the gradual growth of Psora in your patient in this way, from its first manifestation to its present multifariousness, you will find that there are some symptoms that have not thus grown out. How and why such symptoms at all come and remain on, will be explained later.

You will find that these few symptoms have come somehow to be in the patient and that they have remained there without any subsequent development. And these are the symptoms that are unconnected with the main malady, you have to leave them completely out of your account, while making your prescription.

When, however, you have selected the right medicine ignoring these superfluous symptoms, and when your patient will be improving under it, these superfluous symptoms will disappear quite of themselves, as the patient gradually improving, there will be no suitable soil for their existence in him. No new prescribing for the removal of these parasitical symptoms is necessary.

Now, it is necessary for us to ascertain the causes of such symptoms that are like parasites on the parent tree. The first and foremost of these is allopathic medication. The second cause of such superfluous symptoms is at times, an intervening acute disease. If, therefore, there are any acute symptoms in your record, they should also be completely left out of account, while making your prescription.

The difference between acute and chronic prescription is therefore this that, in chronic the medicine has to be miasmatic, while in acute it need not be so.

The stamp of Psora on your patient will suggest all the Anti-Psoric remedies, because the Psoric manifestations are general symptoms, but you will select only one out of all those anti-Psorics has those particulars. Thus, the difference between acute and chronic prescriptions is that, in an acute case any medicine that agrees with the totality of the symptoms of the case can be selected, while in a chronic case, the remedy besides agreeing with the totality of the symptoms must also be anti-miasmatic i.e., anti-psoric, anti-Sycotic or anti-Syphilitic, as the case may be.

Psora, Sycosis and Syphilis that interfere with the normal flow of the life force and lead to abnormal results, and the only way of restoring the life process to its normal course is by administration of a deep acting drug according to the law of similarity. Let us discuss the method of administering drugs on this law.

Before you actually make your selection, you will have to make out the whole array of symptoms into different miasmatic groups, the is to say, if there are all the three miasms Psora, Sycosis and Syphilis in your case, the symptoms that indicate Psora should be placed in one group, the symptoms that indicate Sycosis should be placed in another, and those that indicate syphilis should be placed in a third group.

Then you will have to ascertain as to which of the several miasms is causing the most troubles to your patient at the time of your prescription If it appears that it is Syphilis which is causing the greatest hardship to your patient and the other two miasms Psora and Sycosis, are not predominating for the time being, then you have to select a medicine *on the group of Syphilitic symptoms only.*

The miasms are made predominant one or the other, according as the exciting cause is capable of exciting their manifestations; and it is an inevitable law, that only one miasms is predominant at a time, while the others lie dormant.

The law of prescription in a chronic case is that the medicine indicated by the totality of the symptoms of the miasm predominant will have to be selected and not the medicine indicated by the totality of the symptoms of the whole case. In brief, the prescription must be miasmatic and not otherwise.

If cure is at all to be effected in such cases, the miasms or rather the suppressed manifestation of them, must be made to re-appear, and this re-appearing of suppressed conditions is not possible without the use of high potencies.

COMPLEX MIASMATIC DISEASES[20,6]

If there is only one single miasm, Psora, in a system, there are certain disease symptoms; and if there are two miasms, that is Psora and one only of the other two, sycosis or Syphilis, there are certain more disease symptoms; and if again, there are all the three miasms, there are still more disease symptoms.

These are complexities due to the number of the miasms (uncombined) in the system. But when these miasms exist in the system not merely in number (uncombined), but also in combination, there are still more disease complexities, and these complexities vary according as the combination of two or more miasms.

The system in which Psora combines with the other miasms, gradually gives rise to naughty disease symptoms. Thus, it is the suppression of disease manifestations and combination of miasms, and their number in the said combination that are at the back of all complexities in disease.

Chapter 36

Miasmatic Prescribing[25]

WHEN TO USE MIASMATIC PRESCRIBING

1. *Indicated remedies fail:* When well-selected remedies fail to act, this may indicate the presence of an active miasm, which require treatment with the appropriate nosode. It should of course be remembered that 'well-selected' is a relative term, and the prescription of a nosode in only one of the options that should be considered in the event of a non-response. A 'lack of reaction' has traditionally been considered to be evidence of psoric trait, but in fact any of the miasms seem to be capable of inhibiting the action of indicated remedies.

2. *Patient relapses:* Sometimes the remedy given produces a response in the patient but it is short-lived and is followed by quick return of the patient of his former state. Another possibility is that the symptom picture becomes altered after each prescription but the basic disease tendency is left uncured. Either event may require a nosode in order to bring about fundamental and lasting improvement.

3. *Acute disease fails to resolve:* If an acute disease lingers on and the patient appears to lack the vitality to throw off completely the disease even with the help of indicted remedies, often a nosode will provide the necessary stimulus and clear up the condition. Clarke observed that influenza often seemed to waken up the tubercular miasm, and he found that Tuberculinum Koch was the best remedy to clear up lingering cases. Foubister discovered that both whooping cough and glandular fever could often be cleared up a few doses of *Carcinosin* when they failed to resolve.

4. *Miasm obscures symptom-picture:* Some cases present such an overwhelming miasmatic tendency that it stands out as the dominant feature of the case. In these cases it will sometimes pay dividends to prescribe a nosode as a first remedy, with the expectation that a clearer remedy image will raise and a good response will be obtained when that remedy has been given.

DETERMINING THE DOMINANT MIASM

Just as multiple remedy images are often seen to overlap in the same patient, miasms are seen to do likewise and the art is determining where the emphasis lies at the time of treatment. There are several factor to be taken into account in determining the dominant miasm:

1. *Family history:* When there is a prevalence of certain disease in the ancestors of the patient, this can give clues as to the probable miasmatic inheritance.
2. *Personal medical history:* The pattern of illness throughout a patient's life, including the presenting disorder, can usually be matched to a particular miasmatic disposition.
3. *Remedies which have acted well:* If the remedies to which the patient has previously reacted are all of a similar miasmatic tendency, that miasm is probably predominant. Supposing *Thuja*,

Staphysagria and *Natrium sulphuricum*, have all produced a good response, the sycotic miasm is probably predominant and *Medorrhinum* is likely to be the best indicate nosode.

ACQUIRED MIASMS

So for we have concentrate on inherited disease tendencies, which in practice are those most commonly encountered. It also occurs, however, that a miasm may be acquired during a person's lifetime in one of several ways.

Firstly, following an attack of acute disease, if a chronic disease tendency emerges then an acquire miasm is a possibility. If for example, a person has never regained their health following and attack of chicken-pox, that may be an acquire miasm and will often respond to a dose of the appropriate nosode, which in this case would be Varicella. All of the acute disease nosodes such as a *Morbillinum, Parotidinum, Influenzinum*, etc. may be used in this way Dr. M.L. Tyler made widespread use of these acute disease nosodes in her practice and some remarkable case example are to be found in her writings.

ACTIVITY OF MIASMS

Viewed on a wide scale miasms appear to have cycles of activity, much like epidemics of acute disease, with a prodromal period, a peak and then a decline. Hahnemann noted psora as being predominant, with sycosis and syphilis far less prevalent.

European and American homoeopaths practicing in the late 1800's and early 1900'a observed that the tubercular miasm started to predominate. Following this, the sycotic miasm enjoyed a period of great activity.

In the present day, there is evidence that the cancer miasm is heading towards, a peak of activity, certainly in the so-called 'developed nations', whilst the sycotic and tubercular miasms are still very much in evidence. The syphilitic miasms has been relatively over shadowed throughout this period, yet by no means has it expired completely.

GENETIC DISEASES

If we accept Hahnemann's theory of inherited miasms as being plausible, then all the disorders considered to be 'genetic' by orthodox medicine must be treated as having a miasmatic basis.

Certainly it seems true that children born, for example, with Down's syndrome or cystic fibrosis will invariably have indications for one and usually several nosodes during the course of treatment.

THE USE OF NOSODES

Dr. Fellger said it was absurd to claim that any disease could be cured by its nosode, for after potentizing the nosode, we cannot be satisfied that it is the name condition as when first taken from the diseased individual. It is folly, then, to expect to treat symptoms with its nosode, & the folly is more apparent when we realize that the character of this nosode is essentially changed in the process of potentizing. The only way, therefore, to use a nosode is to prove it on the healthy, like any after drug, & note its symptoms in the regular way.

Some homoeopaths consider that nosodes are no different to any other remedies and that there are no ground for prescribing them other than symptom-similarity. This is a somewhat narrow viewpoint which denies the bulk of clinical experience.

There is abundant evidence that nosodes have certain specific areas of use and that they may be indicated in variety of different ways.

It should also be noted that the nosodes are inadequately represented in the repertories, so that if repertorization is taken as the basic for the prescription then nosode is most unlikely to be prescribed.

The five major miasmatic nosodes are *Psorinum, Medorrhinum, Syphilinum, Tuberculinum* and *Carcinosin*. These are often indicated and prescribed as remedies in their own right, based on the presenting symptom picture. Bearing in mind that they do not feature prominently in the repertories, it is an absolute necessity for the prescribe to become thoroughly acquainted with the nosode remedy pictures.

THE USE OF ANTI-MIASMATIC REMEDIES

All of the deeper acting remedies have been credited with anti-miasmatic properties, ever since Hahnemann recognized the relationship between Psora and Sulphur. It is therefore considered possible to treat on a miasmatic level by employing remedies that are similar to the miasm, as will even instead of to the symptoms.

In Kent's Repertory there no rubrics representing the syphilitic and sycotic miasms but this rubric can be found in the synthetic Repertory of Barthel and Klunnker. The best way to use these rubrics seems to be to take the dominant miasmatic tendency of the patient as the equivalent of one characteristic symptom and to include the corresponding rubric in the repertorization.

SECTION VII: MATERIA MEDICA STUDIES

Chapter 37
Overview

Chapter 38
Psorinum

Chapter 39
Medorrhinum

Chapter 40
Syphilinum

Chapter 41
Tuberculinum

Chapter 42
Carcinosin

Chapter 37

Overview

COMMON MIASMATIC REMEDIES

The lists below are not complete it will give you an idea of the most common remedies and their main miasmatic trait. (Also see the section Introduction to miasms).The concept of remedy-miasm affinities is conjectural and incomplete. You will see from the diagram above that the groups overlap considerably.

ANTI-PSORIC

Abrot. Acet-ac. Agar. Aloe. Alum. Am-br. Ant-c. Anac. Apis. Arg-m. Arg-n. ARS. IOD. Aur. Aur-m. Bar-c. Bell. Benz-ac. Berb. Bor. Bufo. Calc-ac. Calc. Calc-p. Carb-am. Carb-v. Caps. Cist. Clem. Cocc-c. Con. Crot-h. Crot-t. Cup. Dig. Dulc. Ferr. Ferr-p. Fl-ac. Graph. HEP. IOD. Kali-b. Kali-c. Kali-i. Kali-p. Kali-s. Lac-c. LACH. Led. Lyco. Mag-c. Mag-m. Mang. Mez. Mur-ac. Nat-c. NAT-M. Nat-s. Nit-ac. Petr. Phos. Ph-ac. Plat. Plb. PSOR. Pyrc. Sec. Sel. SEP. SIL. Stann. Staph. SULPH. Sul-ac. Taran. TUB.

ANTI-SYCOTIC

Agar. Alumn. Ant-t. Aran. ARG-M. ARG-N. Aster. Aur. Aur-m. Bar-c. bry. Calc. Carbo-an. Calc-s. Carb-v. Caust. Con. Cinnb. Dulc. Ferr. Fl-ac. Graph. Hep-iod. Kal-c. Kali-s. Lach. Lyc. Mang. MED. Merc. Mez. NAT-S. NIT-AC. Petr. Phyt. Puls. Sabin. Sars. Sec. Sel. SEP. Sil. STAPHYS. Sulph. THUJA.

ANTI- SYPHILITICS

Arg-m. Ars. ARS-I. Ars-s-t. Arsat. AUR. AUR-M-N. AUR-M. Bad. Benz-ac. Calc-i. Calc-s. Carb-an. Carb-v. Cinnb. Clem. Con. Cor-r. Crot-h. Fl-ac. Guaj. Hep. iod. Kali-am. Kali-bi. Kali-chl. KALI-I. KALI-S. Lach. Led. MERC-C. MERC-S. MERC-I-F. Mez. MERC-I-R. NIT-AC. Petr. Phos-ac. Phos. PHYTE. Staphys. SIL. Sars. STILL. Sulph. Sulph-i. SYPH. Thuja.

ANTI- TUBERCULAR

Acet-ac. AGAR. aloe alumn. am-c. am-m. ant-ar. ant-t. arg-met. arn. Ars. Ars-i. ars-s-f. arum-t. aur. aur-ar. aur-m. aur-m-n. bac. bac-t. bals-p. Bar-m. berb. beta blatta-o. Brom. Bufo calag. CALC. Calc-i. CALC-P Calc-s. calc-sil. Carb-an. Carb-v. Carbn-s. carc. card-m. cetr. chinin-ar. chlor. coc-c. Con. cur. Dros. Dulc. Elaps erio. eupi. ferr. ferr-ar. Ferr-i. Ferr-p. fl-ac. gad. gad. gal-ac. Graph. Guaj. guajol. ham. helx. HEP. hippoz. ichth. IOD. Kali-ar. kali-bi. KALI-C. Kali-n. Kali-p. KALI-S. kali-sil. Kreos. Lac-d. Lach. lachn. lec. led. LYC. lycps-v. mag-c. mang. Med. Merc. mill. Myrt-c. naphtin. nat-ar. nat-cac. Nat-m. nat-p. nat-s. Nit-ac. Ol-j. ox-ac. petr. Ph-ac. phel. PHOS. pix Plb. PSOR. ptel. PULS. pyrog. rumx. sabal salv. samb. Sang. sarr. SENEC. Seneg. Sep. SIL. slag SPONG. STANN. stann-i. stict. still. sul-ac. sul-i. SULPH. tarent-c. teucr-s THER. thyr. TUB. tub-a. tub-d. verb. ZINC. zinc-i. zinc-p

ANTI- CANCER

Acet-ac. ail. alum. alumn. am-c. Ambr. anan. anil. Ant-m. Apis apoc. arg-met. arg-n. ARS. ars-br. Ars-i. Aster. Aur. Aur-ar. aur-ar. aur-i. Aur-m. aur-m-n. aur-s. Bapt. bar-c. bar-i. bar-met. bell. bism. BROM. Bry. Bufo Cadm-s. Calc. Calc-i. calc-ox. Calc-s. Calen. calth. Carb-ac. CARB-AN. Carb-v. Carbn-s. carc. caust. chel. cholin. Cic. cinnm. Cist. Cit-ac. cit-l. clem. CON. cory. crot-h. Cund. cupr. cupr-act. cupr-f. cur. dulc. elaps eos. epiph. eucal. euph. euph-he. ferr-f. ferr-i. ferr-p. ferr-pic. form. form-ac. fuli. Gali. gent-l. germ-met. Graph. gua. hafn-met. Ham. hep. Hippoz. Hydr. hydrin-m. Iod. Kali-ar. Kali-bi. kali-chl. Kali-cy. Kali-i. Kali-p. Kali-s. Kreos. kres. Lach. lanth-met. Lap-a. lob-e. LYC. maland. matth. med. Merc. merc-c. Merc-i-f. merc-k-i. methyl. Mill. Morph. morph-act. nat-m. nectrin. nicc-met. NIT-AC. Ol-an. Op. orni. oxyg. ph-ac. PHOS. PHYT. pic-ac. polon-met. psor. rab-br. ran-b. rumx-act. Sang. sang. sarcol-ac. scand-met. Scir. sec. sed-r. Semp. sep. sieg. SIL. silphu. sol squil. Syrych-g. sul-ac. Sulph. symph. syph. tarax. tarent-c. tax. Ter. thiosin. Thuj. trif-p. viol-o. visc. X-ray yttr-met. zinc.

Chapter 38

Psorinum[3,4,17,19,22,34,39,40,41,48]

? SCABIES VESICLE

SEROPURULENT MATTER

Appearance:
- Face like inverted pyramid.
- Long pointed nose with big ear.
- Appear unwashed & unclean.
- Dirty dingy crumpled hairs offensive odor
- Unwashable.
- Dry lips especially upper lip swollen; brown black colour of lips with excoriation at the corner of mouth.
- Greasy face & forehead with flush at face.
- Skin rough scaly cracks & fissure it tends to bleed.

MENTALS:
- Gloom, doom, depression.
- 'No way out'.

Psorinum

- Forsaken, restless, sad.
- Self–pity; pessimist; dependent.
- Fears relating to survival [Fear with anxiety; Misfortune; Disease; Something bad will happen].
- Delusion of martyrdom [say all the suffering is good for me].
- Depletion deprivation deficiency [a remedy for poverty (metaphor)].
- Irritable and may suicide [not dramatic means].

GENERALS:
- CHILLY [covers head even in summer].
- Sleep in = Crucifix position.
- Often feel well before illness.
- Under active immune system.
- Recurrent infection.
- Lack of reaction.
- Malabsorption of nutrient.
- Suppression of:
  - Disease
  - Physiological discharge
- Increased appetite in night + in pregnancy.

Food:
- Like Sweets
- Averse to potato; pork; Meat; Fat; Sugar.

Thirst – ++ especially beer.

Perspiration at least exertion offensive odor.

Discharges amelioration.

	Periodicity: very marked 1 weak + 1 day [i.e., 1 day + 8 day + 22 day etc.]
	Matted & prematurely gray hairs.
EYE:	Chronic conjunctivitis / Blephritis / Opthalmia Entropion
EAR:	CSOM
NOSE:	Rhinitis / Sinusitis / Allergy with very strong Periodicity / < Lying back with arms stretched [crucifix].
CHEST:	1. Asthma
	2. Swelling breast
MOUTH:	1. Upper lip swollen dry & cracked/excoriation corner of mouth.
	2. Dry tongue with burnt lip.
	3. Foul breath.
APPETITE:	<< At night << pregnancy << before & after headache.
DIARRHEA:	LOOSE & SPLUTTERY < 1–4 a.m.
G.U.T.:	1. Poor bladder control.
	2. Incontinence on full moon.
	3. Decrease sex desire & Aversion to sex.
	4. Leucorrhoea: Foul & Pours with eruptions.
	5. HOT FLUSH: As if hot water poured over body.
M.S.S.:	Weak joints especially back.
SKIN:	1. Dry & itchy.
	2. Scaly eruptions < winter, > summer.

3. Itching intolerance with despair with burning <wool.
4. Slow healing with lots of suppression.
5. Alteration of dermal & mucousal pathologies.

MODALITY: AGGRAVATION

<<< Cold

< Least draught

< Before stress

< Washing

< Menses

< Winter

< Full moon

<<< Suppression of physiological discharge

< Thunderstorm

< 10 p.m. to 6 a.m.

AMELIORATION

>>> Warmth except skin

> Summer

>> Discharge especially perspiration

> Eating

> Summer

MATERIA MEDICA OF PSORINUM

MIND

- Intolerably self-willed, annoys these about him; a boy suffering from on eruption. – Anxious, full of fear, melancholic; evil forebodings.
- Believes the stitches in heart will Kill him if they do not cease.
- Very depressed, sad, suicidal thoughts.
- Depressed in spirit & hopeless.
- Melancholy after suppressed itch; emaciated, pale, earthy complexion, weakness of limbs; flushes of heat & palpitations prevent sleep; sleep comes toward morning; would like to stay in bed until midday; aversion to work, indifference, weeping seeks solitude, despair of recovery; she is irritable & forgetful.
- Feels the greatest anguish in head, with a whirling before eyes every day, from 5 a.m. until 5 p.m.; walks up & down his room wringing his hands & moaning continually, "on such anguish!" only when he takes his meals he ceases moaning; appetite is good.
- Has been nervous & was obliged to abandon all business; a very disagreeable feeling about head; mental depression; think he will not recover; has lost all hope; can not apply his mind to business;confusion of senses, he can not reckon, attacks of numbness of legs & arms, left side <; < on going to bed; formication & crawling, with pricking & smarting on scalp, & some on extremities; tongue white.

Driven to despair with excessive thinking.

- Disturbances of mind & spirit of all Kinds.

INNER HEAD

- Surging, drawing & digging in forehead < vertigo.
- Pain benumbing over left. Eye & goes to right; < from hour to hour, then diarrhea & nausea, finally bloody vomiting; dizziness, obliges her to lie down; black & blue stars before eyes; veins of temples much distended < and brought on by change of weather, sensitive to touch & pressure of clothes.
- Is always very hungry during headaches.
- Congestion of blood to head immediately after dinner.
- Congestion of head, cheeks & nose red & hot; eruption on face reddens; great anxiety every afternoon after dinner.

OUTER HEAD

- Sensation as if head was separated from body.
- Moist, suppurating, foetid, also dry eruptions on scalp.
- *Taenia capitis.*

Eyes & Sight

- Great photo–phobia, walks with eyes bent upon ground; scurfy eruption on face.
- Lids spasmodically closed; intense photophobia & profuse flow of hot tears; much pustular eruption on face; large brown scab on eye, beneath which pus pours forth abundantly when touched; bowels costive; appetite poor & only for dainties. Pustular Keratitis.
- Right Eye, red internally & externally; vesicle on cornea; eruption on head.

HEARING EARS

- Otorrhoea: < headache; thin ichorous & horrible offensive, like rotten meat; very offensive, purulent (watery, stinking otorrhoea); brown, offensive, from ear; chronic case following scarlet fever.
- Right ear full of crusts & pus, the crusts extended behind auricle to occiput upward upon parietal bone nearly to vertex, forward to right ear & over cheek; upon edge of region involved small vesicles filled with clear fluid, which become yellow, then crusted, & pus flowed from beneath crusts.
- Scurfs on ears, & humid scurfs behind ear.

NOSE SMELL

- Dry coryza with stoppage of nose.
- Septum inflamed, with, suppurating pustules.
- Bloody, purulent discharge from nose
- Chronic catarrh; dropping from posterior nares, so as to awake him at night; hawking quantities of lumpy mucus gave temporary relief from feeling of fullness; mucous in nose would dry like white dry like white of egg, needed to be forcibly removed.
- Pain in liver, < from sneezing.

FACE

- Painful tension & pressure in right zygoma, towards ear.
- Pain as if lame condyle of jaw.
- Sweat of face with severe heat.
- Moist scab behind ears with Dry tetter on back of head, on both cheeks extending up ward to eyes & down ward to corners of mouth, reddish, dry pimples, < frequent loose stool.

- An offensive-smelling, crusty eruption extending over whole face, had completely closed eyes.
- Eruption on face; whole face covered with a crust, lips & eyelids swollen, aversion to light, large moistening spots on head & behind ears.

TEETH & GUMS

- Looseness of teeth; they feel so loose, fears they may fall.

THROAT

- Sensation of a plug or lump in throat impending hawking.
- Tooth burns, feels scalded.
- Tension & swollen feeling in throat.
- Cutting tearing pain in throat on swallowing.
- Steam arising from fat causes immediate constriction of throat & chest.

THIRST

- Thirst: during dinner; with dryness of throat; especially for beer, mouth feels so dry.

EATING & DRINKING

- Immediate after dinner, congestion of blood to head.
- Pain in chest extending to shoulder < after cold drinks.

HICCOUGH, BELCHING, NAUSEA, VOMITING

- Eructations: sour, rancid; tasting & smelling like rotten eggs; room is filled with a very offensive odour (*Arn., Graph., Ant.-t.*)

- *Arn.*– especially in a.m., *Ant-t;* At night; *Graph.;* In a.m. only, after rising, disappearing on rinsing the mouth.
- Waterbrash when lying down, > on getting up.

STOMACH

- Weakness of stomach.
- Frequent oppression of stomach, especially after eating.

HYPOCHONDRIA

- Deep–seated sticking, pressing pain in region of liver, < from external pressure & lying on right side; pain hinders sneezing, laughing, yawning, coughing, deep inspiration & walking.

ABDOMEN

- Flatulence with disorders of liver.
- Colic: removed by eating; > passing foetid flatus.

STOOL & RECTUM

- Semiliquid, brownish, insufferably nasty; passed during sleep, with undigested food. Infantile diarrhea.
- Horribly offensive, nearly painless, almost involuntary, dark & watery stool; only at night & most toward morning.
- Involuntary stool during sleep.
- Haemorrhage from rectum; with constipation.

URINARY ORGANS

- Involuntary urine, can not hold it; vesical paresis. Typhus.
- Scanty urination nearly every half hours, with burning in urethra.

- Condylomata.

MALE SEXUAL ORGAN

- After suppressed gonorrhea; rheumatism, lameness; conjunctivitis, with granulation; intense photophobia to light.
- Chronic Gleet.
- Sycotic excrescences on edges of prepuce, with itching burning.
- Hydrocoele, caused by repeated inflammation, in consequence of pressure from a truss.

FEMALE SEXUAL ORGANS

- Left ovary indurate after a violent knock; fallowed by itching eruption on body & face.
- Knotty lump above right groin; even a bandage hurts.
- Metrorrhagia.
- Amenorrhoea: In psoric subjects when tetter is covered by thick scurfs; with phthisis.
- Dysmenorrhoea near climaxis.
- Menstrual disorders during climaxis.
- Leucorrhoea, large lumps, unbearable in odour; violent pains in sacrum & right loin; great debility.

PARTURITION PREGNANCY LACTATION

- Mammae swollen, painful; redness of nipples, burning around them.
- Pimples itching violently, about nipples; oozing a fluid during pregnancy.
- Mammary Cancer.

LARYNX & TRACHEA

- Voice weak & trembling.

RESPIRATION

- Convalescents go out for a walk, instead of being invigorated return home in order to get breath or to lie down so they breathe more easily, feel < instead of > from being in open air.

- Dyspnoea: < when sitting up to write,> when lying down, Congestion to head after dinner, great despondency; < the nearer arms are brought to body.

COUGH

- Severe, dry cough with oppression of chest & pain as if everything in chest were raw & scathed; fever in evening; great depression of spirits, making life burdensome to him.

- Cough, causing tearing from center of chest to throat all on right side; cough < at night; urine escapes when coughing.

- Dry cough, Pain in chest for last three month, a constricting pressure at fourth & fifth ribs near sternum, excessive irritability & ill humor.

- Cough < expectoration; asthma, thinks he will die.

- Cough with salty tasting, green & yellow expectoration; oppression of chest; gradual loss of strength after suppressed itch.

- Cough aggravates pain in liver & pain in chest extending to shoulder.

INNER CHEST & LUNGS

- Pain in chest, as if raw, as from subcutaneous ulceration.

- Stitches: in sternum, with backache; from behind forward in chest & back when breathing; in rt. side of chest when breathing.
- Fixed pain in right side of chest.
- Chest pain from coughing.
- Heat sensation in chest.
- Tedious recovery in pneumonia.
- Pain in chest grow more severe two or three times a day, begins with chilliness & trembling, followed by heat; great anxiety of heart & mind with fear of death, dyspnoea & restlessness; attacks passes off with sour, clammy sweat & chilliness; sweat however occurs every night independent of attack.
- Dull pressure in right side of chest, extending thence, over whole chest, < bending forward in writing, not by motion or deep inspiration; dry cough & expectoration of lumps of mucus; speaking effects him very much; great prostration after preaching, so that he must rest a long time to recuperate; voice is not husky but it requires all his strength to get through with his word; chest narrow, shoulders projected. Phthisis.

HEART

- Gurgling in region of heart, particularly noticeable when lying.
- Rheumatic pericarditis; pulse 144; skin dry; pain in head & limbs but more particularly in shoulder; dyspnoea, with pain in region of heart; effusion, indistinct heart sounds; murmur with first sound; inability to lie down.

NECK & BACK

- Herpetic eruption on side of neck extending from cheek.
- Nape of neck excoriated by discharge from eczema capitis.
- Constricting and pressing pain in small of back; < from motion.

- Backache when walking, with stitches in sternum.
- Backache with constipation.
- Spina bifida.

UPPER LIMB

- Tearing in arms.
- Tetter on arms small millet like eruption exuding a yellow fluid; itches intensely in heat.
- Itching eruption on wrist with tearing in limbs.
- Dry tetter on wrists with rheumatism in limbs.
- Swelling & tension of backs of hands & of fingers.
- Copper colored eruption or red blisters on back of hand.
- Nails brittle.

LOWER LIMBS

- Sciatica
- Purpura on inner side of thigh
- Old itch eruption on inner side of thigh and in popliteal space.
- Knees give way under him.
- Dry herpes, especially in bend of knees.
- Eruption about joints makes walking difficult, as if encased in armour.
- Vesicles becoming ulcers, on feet.
- Large swelling about ankle.
- Feeling when walking as if left foot were pulled around inward. Locomotor ataxia.
- Scars between second and third toes of left Foot.

- Gout in lower extremities.
- Hands & feet feel as if broken early in morning and after a little work.
- Chronic rheumatism in limbs, with a dry eruption on wrists.
- Arthritis: rheumatism, especially in chronic forms.
- Long standing gout pains etc; dry cough; constrictive pressure and cutting, tearing pain at sternum near fourth and fifth ribs; greatest despondency and ill humour.
- Hands moist, with cold, clammy sweat, the very touch of which was unpleasant; Profuse sweating of feet; feet very painful, causing shuffling gait.
- Caries; rachitis.

NERVES

- Ennui tedium.
- Very weak and miserable after suppressed itch.
- Trembling and chilliness, with attacks of pain in chest.
- Debility: independent of any organic disease; loss of appetite; tendency to perspiration on exertion and at night
- Constantly increasing debility, with abdominal affections.

SLEEP

- Child apparently well, but at night would twist and turn and fret from bedtime till morning and next day be as lively as ever.
- Sick babies will not sleep at night, but worry, fret and cry.
- In morning lies in same position as when he fall asleep.

FEVER

- When walking a walk profuse sweat with consequent debility, taking cold easily.
- Profuse sweating relieves all the complaints; chronic disorder
- After malaria colour of face worse.

TISSUES

- Thinner than usual, pale, exhausted
- Great emaciation, in children; they are pale, delicate, sickly, will not sleep day or night, but worry, fret and cry, or child is good, play all day, is restless, troublesome, screaming all night.
- Glandular swellings with eruption on head.
- All excretions, diarrhoea, leucorrhoea, menstrual flow and perspiration, have a carrion like odour.
- Body has a filthy smell even after the bath
- Whole body painful, easily sprained and hurts himself
- Rheumatism and arthritis
- Deeply penetrating ichorous ulcers.
- Carries; rachitis; dropsy
- The joints are easily sprained or strained.
- Increasing disposition to strains and to overlift oneself even at a very slight exertion of the muscles, even in slight mechanical work, in reaching out or stretching for something high up, in lifting things that are not heavy, in quick turns of he body, pushing, etc. such a tension of stretching of the muscles often then occasions long confinement to bed, all grades of hysterical troubles, fever, Haemoptysis etc. While person who are not psoric lift such burdens as their muscles are able to, without the slightest after effects.

- The joints are easily sprained at any false movement.
- In the joint of foot there is pain or trauma as if it would break.
- Softening of bones, curvature of spine (deformity, hunch back), curvature of long bones of thighs and legs (morbus, anglicus, rickets)
- Fragility of the bones.

SKIN

- Skin has a dirty, dingy look, as if patient never washed; in some places looks coarse as if bathed in oil, sebaceous.
- Scaly condition of skin of whole body; skin has a dirty, tawny colour, although carefully kept; much itching causing desire to scratch, which gave but temporary relief; some months back, instead showed signs of eruption, which soon became a thick, dirty looking marks of scales and pus, painful and violently itching; at time pain kept her awake at night.
- Eczema behind ears, on scalp and in bends of elbows and armpits, accompanied by abscesses affecting bones; nothing relieved, but the eruption disappeared, to reappear again, years after, on wrists, there was then a patch on each wrist as large as a half dollar, with intense itching, preventing sleep, with constant desire to scratch.
- Itch: dry on arms and chest, most severe on finger joints; followed by boils; inveterate cases with symptoms of tuberculosis; in recent cases, with eruptions in bends of elbows and around wrists; repeated outbreak of single pustules after main eruption seems all gone.
- Psoriasis; Psoriasis syphilitica.
- Pustules or boils on head, particularly on scalp; scalp had a dirty look and emitted an offensive odour; fine, red eruption, forming small white scales; pustules on hands.

- Burning, itching pustules after vaccination.
- Retrocession of eruption, Measles.
- Suppressed eruption.

WHEN TO USE PSORINUM

- Especially adapted to the psoric constitution.
- In chronic cases when well selected remedies fail to relieve or permanently improve (in acute diseases, *Sulph*); when *Sulph*. Seems indicated but fails to act.
- Lack of reaction after severe acute disease. Appetite will not return.
- Children are pale, delicate, sickly. Sick babies will not sleep day or night but worry, fret, cry (*Jalap*); child is good, plays all day; restless, troublesome, screaming all night (rev. of *Lyco*.).
- Great weakens & debility; from loss of animal fluids; remaining after acute disease; independent of or without any organic lesion, or apparent cause.
- Body has filthy smell, even after bathing.
- The whole body painful, easily sprained & injured.
- Great sensitiveness to cold air or change of weather.
- Stormy weather he feels acutely; feels restless for days before or during a thunderstorm (*Phos*); dry, scaly eruptions; never recovered from typhoid.
- Feels unusually well day before attack.
- Extremely psoric patient; nervous, restless, easily startled.
- All excretions:– Diarrhoea, Leucorrhoea, Menses, Perspiration have a carrion like odour.
- Anxious, full of fear; evil forebodings.

- Religious melancholy; very depressed, sad suicidal thoughts; despair of salvation (*Med.*), of recovery.
- Despondent; fear he will die; that he will fail in business; during climaxis; making his own life & that of those about him intolerable.
- Driven of despair excessive itching.
- Headache; preceded by flickering before eyes; by dimness of vision or blindness (*Lac.d., Kali-bi*); by black spots or rings.
- Headache; always hungry during; > while eating (*Anac., Kali-p*); from suppressed eruptions, or suppressed menses; by nosebleed (*Med.*)
- Hair; dry, lusterless, tangles easily, glues together (*Lyc.*), Plica polonica (*Borax, Sars, Tub.*).
- Scalp; dry, scaly or moist, foetid, suppurating eruptions; oozing a sticky, offensive fluid (*Graph., Mez.*)
- Intense photophobia, with inflamed lids; can not open the eyes; lies with face buried in pillow. (*Con*)
- Ears; humid scurf's & soreness on & behind ears; oozing & offensive viscid fluid (*Graph*)
- Otorrhoea; thin ichorous, horribly foetid discharge, like decayed meat; chronic after measles or scarlatina.
- Acne; all forms, simplex, rosacea; <during menses from coffee, fat sugar, meat; when the best selected remedies fails or not palliates.
- Hungry in the middle of night; must have thing to eat (*Cina, Sulph*).
- Eructation's tasting of rotten eggs (*Arn, Ant-t., Graph.*)
- Quinsy; tonsils greatly swollen; difficult, painful swallowing; burns, feels scalded; cutting, tearing, intense pain to ear on swallowing (Painless – *Bar-c.*); profuse, offensive saliva; tough

mucus in throat, must hawk continually. To not only > acute attack but eradicate the tendency.

- Hawk up cheesy balls, size of a pea of disgusting taste & carrion like odour (*Kali-m*)

- Diarrhea; sudden imperative (*Aloe, Sulph*); stools watery, dark brown, foetid; smells like carrion; involuntary at night from 1 to 4 AM; after severe acute disease; teething in children; when weather changes.

- Constipation; obstinate, with backache; from inactivity of rectum; when sulphur fail to relieve.

- Enuresis; from vesicle paresis; during full moon, obstinate cases, with a family history of eczema.

- Chronic gonorrhea of years duration that can neither be suppressed nor cured; the best selected remedies fails.

- Leucorrhoea; large, clotted lumps of on intolerable odour; violent pain in sacrum; debility; during climaxis.

- During pregnancy; most obstinate vomiting, fetus moves too violently; when the best selected remedy fails to relive; to correct the psoric diathesis of the unborn.

- Profuse perspiration after acute disease, with relief of all sufferings (*Calad, Nat-m.*)

- Asthma, dyspnoea; <in open air sitting up (*Laur*); >lying down & Keeping arms stretched for apart (rev of *Ars.*) despondent thinks he will die.

- Cough returns every winter.

- Hay fever; appearing regularly every year the same day of the month; with asthmatic, psoric or eczematous history patient should be treated the previous winter to eradicate the diathesis & prevent summer attack.

- Cough; after suppressed itch, or eczema; chronic of yearly duration; marked on waking & evening on lying down (*Phos.*, *Tub*) sputter green yellow or salty mucus; pus like coughs a long time before expectorating.
- Abnormal tendency to receive skin disease (*Sulph.*) eruptions, early suppurate (*Hep.*); dry, inactive, rarely sweats; dirty look, as if never washed; coarse, greasy, as if bathed in oil; bad effects from suppressed by sulphur or zinc ointments.
- Sleepless from intolerable itching; or frightful dreams of robbers, danger etc (*Nat-m.*)
- Psorinum should not be given for psora or psoric diathesis, but like every other remedy, upon a strict individualization. The totality of symptoms and then we realize it wonderful work.

RELATIONS

- Antidoted by coffee, *Nux-v.* (if < when too frequently repeated or over dose)
- Compatible: *Carb-v.*, Cinchona, opium, *Sulph.*, *Tub.* (if want of susceptibility to medicinal action)
- Followed well by *Alum., Bar., Hep., Lyc., Sulph., Tub.*
- Complimentary: *Sulph., Tub.*, after *Lact. Ac. & Nux-v.* (Vomiting of pregnancy); after *Arn., Bellis, Ham.*, (In traumatic affections of the ovaries); *Sulph* follow *Psor.* in mammary cancer.
- Inimical: *Apis, Crot, Lach* & the serpent poisons.
- Compare: Cham: *Jalap* (sick babies, fret day & night); (happy all day, screams at night) (*Lyc.*) cry all day, sleeps at night. − Nervous effects of electric storms (*Phos, X–ray*).
- *Gels., Lac-d, Kali-bi,* (headache Preceded by dim vision & dark spote); *Anac., Kali-p* (headache with hunger > while eating); *Meli.* (Headache relived by noses bleed).

- *Bar-c., Lyc. Sars, Tub.* (Plica Polonica). – *Kali-mur.* (offensive, cheesy balls from the throat).
- *Calc., Nat-m.* (all symptoms> by lying down & keeping arms stretched for apart; (*Ars*; must it up & lean forward).
- *Phos, Tub.* (cough & affections of the respiratory tract < morning on waking, & evening when lying down);
- *Graph., Hep., Sil.,* (eruptions & slight injuries of the skin easily suppurating).
- *Dig.* (drinking<cough)–*Bry., Nat-m* (sallow, greasy face).
- *Puls., Tub.* (erratic shifting pains< from fats & pastry < evening).
- *Sang., Tub.,* (sensation as if tongue were burned).
- *Ars., Bapt., Pyr.* (Sensation as if parts were separated, *Ars.* Body at waist, *Bapt.* Brain & limbs).
- *Kali-c., Pyr., Tub.* (Profuse sweat during convalescence).
- *Ambr., Caps, Cina, Laur, Op, Valer.* (lack of susceptibility to best selected remedy).
- *Gels., Kali-iod, Sab., Cin.n.* (hay fever).
- *Cina, China-s, Ign., Lyc., Sulph., Tub.* (hungry at night, can't sleep until they eat).
- *Ars., Rhus, X–ray, Tub.,* causes: mental emotions, or mental labour; over lifting; suppressed eruptions; weather changes, electric storms; traumatism; sprains & dislocations.

Chapter 39

Medorrhinum[3,4,17,19,34,39,41,48]

Purulent pus of untreated gonorrhea.

SYSTEM AFFINITY:

1. Genito Urinary
2. Mucosae & Skin
3. Joints
4. Lungs
5. Nervous tissue

MENTALS:

- DUALITY [*Diplococcus*].
- Basic conflict Good vs Devil.
- Taint with extremes of pathology & personality.
- People of the night.
- Seek sensual & pleasure principle.
- Are cruel, hard, passionate people extremist in temperament.
- Addicted to drugs & alcohol.

- Desire to experience every thing
- Excess of everything
- Extreme fluctuation of mood & behaviour
- Eventually overcome by shame. [THE SYCOTIC SHAME] [*Thuja* = Shame covered up; *Med.* = Shame expressed]

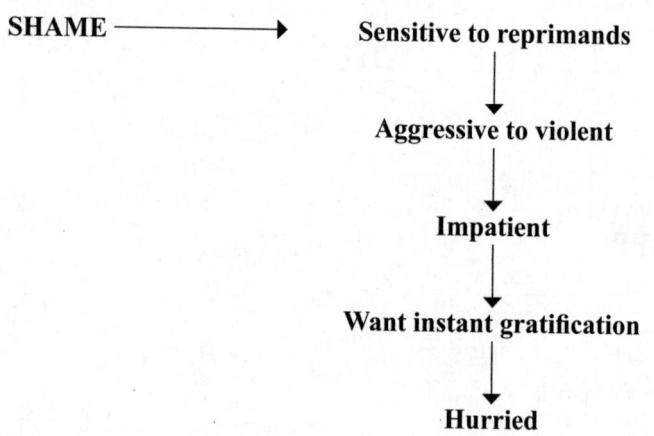

SHAME ⟶ Sensitive to reprimands ↓ Aggressive to violent ↓ Impatient ↓ Want instant gratification ↓ Hurried

DUALITY:

Love passionately ⟶ Jealous ⟶ Suspicious ⟶ Hate

Love Animals ⟶ but are cruel to them.

Concentration very clear or foggy.

Delusion: Someone is behind them.

Fear: Especially about mental health.

Often very weepy; while telling their sign & symptoms.

Often found biting nails / restless legs.

Hypersensitive to environmental change / clairvoyant.

SYCOTIC TRIAD:

- << Damp.
- Green discharge especially catarrh.
- Warts.

AILMENT FROM ABUSE OF:

- Oral pills
- Steroids
- Antibiotics
- Vaccination

APPEARANCE:

- Full body; Large full lips; Greasy skin; Dandruff; Bushy eye brows; Coarse facial appearance; extreme sycosis = Downs syndrome.

MODALITIES:

- >> Sea.
- >> Night & better evening [*Med./Aur.*].
- << Damp.
- Food Desire unripe fruit/sweet/ice cream/fat/desire but worse by oranges/chocolate/averse Chinese food/slimy food.
- Thirst ++ for cold drinks.
- Fluid retention.
- Multiple fungal infection.
- Soft tissue tumors.

HEAD:

- Pain deep boring in middle of the head [deep]
- Pulls hair in pain.

EYES:

- Clear yellow discharge; eyes shock in morning.
- Reiter's syndrome.
- Gritty eye / visual disturbances.

EARS:

CSOM (Chronic Suppurative Otitis Media).

NOSE:

Chronic Rhinitis / Sinusitis / Post nasal catarrh.

THROAT:

Always clearing his throat.

CHEST:

Bronchiectasis / Pleurisy / etc.

GIT (GASTRO INTESTINAL SYSTEM:

- Early dental decay [D/d *Staph., Merc., Kreos., Thuja*].
- Peptic ulcer [*Med.* wakes at 2 a.m. with pain]
- Constipation easier to expel bending backwards [especially in children].

CVS (CARDIOVASCULAR SYSTEM):

- Early age MI
- Increased cholesterol
- Cardiomyopathy

GU (GENITO-URINARY SYSTEM):

- All possible pathologies.
- Including strictures [D/d *Thios., Clem., Sil., Carc., Graph., Tub.*].
- Polycystic ovary / endometriosis / unexplained infertility / hypo or hypergonadism / sexual precocity / Impotence.
- Very high libido may lead to perversion: homosexuality.
- Masturbation in children [*Med.; Bufo; Plat.; Staph.; Carc.*].

ENDOCRINE SYSTEM:

Hypo / Hyper function.

MUSCULO-SKELETAL SYSTEM:

- Acute / Chronic rheumatism stitches insoles, as if walking on pebbles.
- Burning feet stick out of covers.
- > Walking on cold floor.
- Feels as if walking on stones.
- Oedema [Ankle swelling].
- Ankylosing spondylosis [*Med.*].

SLEEP:

- Genu-pectoral position
- Lascivious dreams / dreams of drinking.

SKIN:

- Eczema.
- Warts.
- Fungal infection.
- Cutaneous tumors.
- Aggressive urticaria.

- Nappy rash with demarcated edge [*Med.*].

GENERALS:

- Family History of Congenital heart disease.
- Family History of Early age MI.
- Sudden precipitation of serious illness.
- Backward & defective children.
- Down's [First remedy to think of].
- Brain damage.
- Memory problem [All rubrics].

MATERIA MEDICA OF MEDORRHINUM

MIND

- Indisposed to work or make mental effort; desire for rest and dread of change; noise, confusion, disorderliness of surroundings, depression and much anxiety, especially after sleep; irritable if the room is not lighted enough to make everything distinct; craving for stimulants, but cannot endure the effects, for they cause a wild, crazy feeling in brain after the first sleep; same effect from closing eyes.

- Usually depressed; easily tired; disinclined to any exertion, & yet unable to keep still; forgetful; unable to think connectedly; mind wanders from subject, even in reading; can't think at all if hurried.

- Always wakens tired in the morning; hates to do anything that must be done, even nice things; gets nervous & excited about riding & driving as soon as the time is fixed.

- Constant state of anguish. Always a feeling of impending danger, but knows not what. There is no cause for such feelings, as she

- is not obliged to do anything when disinclined; is situated that nothing need cause her trouble.
- Inability to think continuously, to talk or to listen to talking when weary; vacant feeling in head.
- Forgetful, can't remember the least thing any length of time; writes everything down of any importance; can't trust herself to remember it; greatly irritability & disgust with life.
- The impatience, excitement, wild feelings; the unreal, dazed condition; the gloom & fear in the dark; the difficulty of speaking without tears, are marked evidence of functional derangement of the nervous system.
- Medorrhinum is forgetful of names, words etc. but instead of like *Syphilinum*, it forgets what it is reading, even to the last line read; it can't concentrate its attention; thinks words spelled wrong & have no meaning, etc.
- It develops a peculiar sensitivity especially in relation to occurrences affecting itself.
- It feels the evil coming to it, & the bad news before it arrives, of course it is selfish, & it is easily hurt by a harsh word.
- It is also introspective, self-accusative, remorseful. Time moves slowly to it, therefore it is hurried.
- We find a dazed condition from the loss of thread of thought, which annoys & causes a dread of saying the wrong thing, & a difficulty in stating symptoms.
- It is always anticipating, fearing evil will happen, loss of reason or suicide.
- It fears it has committed the unpardonable sin & cares little for the result, because of the sinking, restless, uneasy, unbalanced nerves.
- Feeling of desperation; did not care if he went to heaven or hell.
- Great weakness of memory.

- Dullness of memory & desire to procrastinate, because business seemed so lasting, or as if it never could be accomplished.
- Forgetful of names, letters of words & initial letters.
- Cannot remember names; has to ask names of her most intimate friends; forgets her own.
- Time moves too slowly.
- Dazed feeling; a far off sensation, as though thing done today occurred a week ago.
- Loses threads of her talk.
- In conversation he would occasionally stop, & on resuming make remark that he could not think what word he wanted to use.
- Seems to herself to make wrong statements, because she does not know what to say next, begins all right but does not know to finish weight on vertex, which seems to affect mind.
- Great difficulty in stating her symptom & has to be asked over again.
- One sight saw large people in room; large rats running felt a delicate hand smoothing her head from front to back.
- Fear he is going to die.
- Sensation as if all life was unreal like a dream.
- Wild & desperate feeling, as of incipient insanity.
- Cannot speak without crying.
- Is in a great hurry; when doing anything is in such hurry that she gets fatigued.
- In always anticipating; feels most matters sensitively before they occur & generally correctly.
- Anticipates death.
- Dread of saying wrong thing when she has headache
- Everything startles her, news coming to her seems to touch her heart before she hears it.
- Wake at an early hour with a frightened sensation, as if something dreadful had happened; heavy weight & great heat

in head; could not rest in bed; felt as if she has to do something to rid her mind of this torture.
- Fear of dark.
- Cross through day, exhilarated at night, wants to play.
- Irritated at little thing.
- Very impatient.

HEAD

- Intense itching of scalp.

EYES & SIGHT

- Feeling as if she stares at everything, as if eyes protruded.
- Aching in eyeball, Pressing & heat in vertex a tendency to shut eyes.
- Neuralgic pain in eyeballs; when pressing eyelids together; < when rolling them.
- Continuous watering of eyes, great heat & sensation of sand under lids.
- Feeling of pain & irritation, & sensation of sticks in eyes, lids & especially inner canthi, redness & dryness of lids, congestion of sclerotic & sensation of a cool wind blowing in eyes, especially inner canthi.
- Ptosis of outer end of both upper Lids, particularly requiring exertion to open them.
- Swelling of upper lids; soreness & smarting of edges.
- Decided tendency to irritation of edges of lids.
- Pulling pain in left lower lid from outer canthus.

EARS & HEARING

- Partial or transient deafness; pulsation in ears
- Hardness of hearing.

NOSE & SMELL

- Epistaxis.

FACE

- Great pallor; yellowness of, particularly around eyes, as if occurring from a bruise (greenish yellow); yellow.
- Neuralgia of right upper & lower jaw, extending to temples.
- Tendency to stiffness in jaws & tongue.
- Rigidity of muscles of face, especially of lower lip, drawing it up Right to teeth; jaws stiff, unable to open them; deglutition nearly impossible; throat filled by saliva.

TEETH & GUMS

- Teeth have serrated edges, or are chalky & easily decay (*Syph.*; teeth are cupped, decayed at edges tooth gone since four years; intense neuralgic pains extending to whole head, causing sleeplessness; severe pains all over head, with external heat.
- Pale gums.

MOUTH

- Very sore mouth, ulcers on tongue & in buccal cavity, like blisters.
- Blisters on inner surface of lips & cheeks, skin peeling off in patches.

APPETITE, THIRST, DESIRES, AVERSIONS

- Violent retching & vomiting; first glairy mucous, then frothy & watery, & lastly coffee grounds; accompanied by intense headache, with great despondency & sensation of impending death; during paroxysm was continuously praying.

- Great craving for salt.

STOMACH

- Sensation in pit of stomach as of a paper of pins that seemed to force themselves through flesh, drawing her to rise & double up & scream; pins seem to come from each side. Abscess of liver.
- Cramps in stomach as from wind.
- Intense pain in stomach & up. abdomen, with a sensation of tightness.
- Bilious colic with frequent vomiting & nausea; diarrhoeic stools, chilliness & perspiration on face & neck.
- Congestion of liver.
- Grasping pain in liver & spleen.
- Burning heat around the back, like a coal of fire. Abscess of liver.
- Severe pain from abscess extending to rt. shoulder & down elbow.
- Throbbing & thumping in region of suprarenal capsule, seeming to come from abscess or sore spot just below fifth rib, right side; creeping chills in region of rt. kidney, throbbing, contracting, drawing & relaxing as if caused by icy cold insects with claws.

ABDOMEN

- Intense agonizing pain in solar plexus; surface cold; eructation tasting sulphurated hydrogen pit of stomach.
- Ascites; abdomen greatly distended; palpation showed water; urine very scanty & high coloured.

STOOL & RECTUM

- White diarrhoea.
- Can only pass stool by leaning very for back; very painful, as if there was a lump on posterior Surface of sphincter; so painful as to cause tears.
- Constriction & inertia of bowels with ball like stools.
- Running from anus greenish yellow, thin horribly offensive stools.
- Child with great emaciation, diarrhoea green, watery, slimy, yellow, curdled, like boiled potatoes chopped up with greens, thin cream colored, watery, smelling like rotten eggs; stools passes involuntarily; apparently lifeless, except that it rotates head on pillow.
- Painful attacks of piles, not bleeding, hot swelling of left side of anus; pin worms.

URINARY ORGANS

- Pain in renal region, profuse urination relieves.
- Very distinct bubbling sensation in right kidney; sensation of three bubbles in right renal region, moving like bubbling in water, causing faintness; deathly feeling in kidneys, with great depression of spirit, similar to effect of cold setting in renal region, prostration after urination.
- Urine high coloured.
- Strong smelling urine.
- Urine covered with a thick greasy pellicle.
- Nocturnal urination entirely ceased, the chamber empty in morning.
- Painful tenesmus of bladder & bowels when urinating.

- Passes an enormous quantity of high coloured, strong smelling urine in bed every night; thinks it is in after part of night, as he is always wet in the morning; overwork & too muck heat or being in cold, aggravates this condition.
- Diabetic condition; profuse & frequent urination.

MALE SEXUAL ORGAN – IMPOTENCE

- Gonorrhoeal flow thin, transparent, mixed with opaque whitish mucus, stains linen yellow.
- Intense & frequent erections day & night.
- Pains along urethra while urinating, drawing burning.
- Burning in meatus during urination, & a feeling of soreness through whole urethra; also after urinating a feeling as if something more remained in urethra.
- Scanty, yellowish, gleety discharge, of many months standing, showing most plainly in morning, gumming up orifice.
- Profuse, yellow, purulent discharge from urethra, most copious in morning.
- Cannot retain urine more than an hour, after 5 or 6 p.m.
- Cannot retain urine through night.
- Gleety, gonorrheal discharge, stains clothes a dirty brown, discharges extremely slow, at times it lakes half an hour to empty bladder, leaving him in a weak condition; during urination, painful rectal tenesmus; chilliness when bladder is too full, > by urination; if he urinates after getting warm in bed, has to urinate every hour rest of night; faint, indefinite sense of chillness, followed by frequent calls to urinate, urine being hot, copious & followed by spinal chill & incontinence of urine on getting cold.

FEMALE SEXUAL ORGAN – GREAT SEXUAL DESIRE AFTER MENSES

- Ulceration of neck of uterus, which looks ragged & torn, inflamed & covered with stringy pus; had gonorrhoea.
- Menses very dark; stains difficult to wash out.
- After very profuse menses, neuralgia in paroxysms in head with twitching & drawing in limbs & cords of neck, which were like wires; pain in lower abdomen, with profuse, yellowish leucorrhoea.
- Membranous dysmenorrhoea Menses was accompanied by terrible pains of a grinding character. Flow scanty, & on the second day there was a passage of a firmly organized membrane. The mental symptom was a constant feeling as if something was behind her. She could not get away from that sensation. It was of nothing definite, simply something terrible behind her, peeping over her shoulder, causing her to look around anxiety.

LARYNX TRACHEA & BRONCHIA

- Choking caused by a weakness or spasm of epiglottis, could not tell which; larynx stopped so that no air could enter only > by lying on face & protruding tongue. (*Acet-ac.*)
- Dryness of glottis very annoying, with pain during deglutition; great hoarseness.
- Bronchial catarrh spreading into larynx; swelling of tonsils & glands of throat extended also into ears causing transient deafness.

COUGH

– Cough, < on lying down,> lying on stomach.

– Cough, < at night causing retching.

CHEST

– Pain in right shoulder as though it came from light, straight through.

– Constricted sensation at bottom of both lungs; finally dull, heavy pain at top of left lung.

– Awful pains, in phthisis, in middle lobes.

– Incipient consumption.

HEART

– Feeling of a cavity where heart ought to be.

NECK & BACK

– Pain straight through from left to right shoulder.

– Heat in medulla & spine.

– Throbbing & thumping in region of right suprarenal capsule seeming to come from a abscess or sore spot just below fifth rib, right side, under breast; creeping chills in region of rt kidney, throbbing contracting drawing & relaxing; as if caused by icy cold insects with claws. Abscess of liver.

– Pain in lumbar portion of spine; myalgic; induration of testes

– Lumbago caused by straining in lifting

UPPER LIMBS

- Rheumatic pain in right shoulder & arm.
- Severe pain from abscess, extending to right shoulder & down to elbow.
- Pain commencing under left scapula running down left arm to little finger, which pricked as if asleep.
- Consumptive incurvation of nails (Clubbing).

LOWER LIMBS

- Rheumatic pains in muscles of legs.
- Kind of cramp in calf at night, muscles knotted, > stretching; not cramp, but knotting.
- Sudden intense pain in left ankle, back of joint, on going to bed, could not move limb or body without screaming; could find no position of comfort.
- Burning of feet, wants them uncovered & fanned.
- Swelling & itching in soles, itching between toes, & pulling pains extending up to knees; itching, painful, papular eruption around waist, & hive like eruption wherever flush is pushed on.
- Tenderness of soles so that he could not stand on them at all & had to walk on his knees.
- Soreness in ball of foot under toes.
- Cold & sweaty, < during winter.
- Old foot sweats, < during winter,
- Almost entire loss of nervous force in legs & arms; exhausted by slightest effort.
- Pain like rheumatism along right side, right hip, left leg (up, lower left); pains drawing, < in dampness, lt. leg swollen near knee.

- Stiffness throughout body & joints.
- Deformity of finger joints, large, puffy knuckles, swelling, stiffness & pain of both ankles; great tenderness of heels & balls of feet; the swellings of all affected joints were puffy like wind falls; general condition worse inland near shore.

NERVES

- Consumptive languor; great general depression of vitality.
- Very tired.

SLEEP

- Wakeful; slept toward morning.
- Becomes wide awake at 6 p.m., & continues so till 12, with entire passivity of brain & cessation of thought; slight restlessness.

FEVER

- Great burning heat all over body, with flashes of heat in face & neck.
- Profuse sweat about neck
- Chill commencing from 3–4 p.m.; chill with headache, thirst, nausea, some times vomiting; fever with headache, thirst, nausea, principally on head & neck; pains from waist downwards; frequent urination, dark colour; frequent, tasteless eructation; constipation; bad taste in mouth in morning.
- Chill commenced in small of back, running up & down, & as it ceased, profuse & frequent urination appeared & continuous during fever, congestion of chest simulating pneumonia during fever, causing great alarm; great renal distress during paroxysms; thirst during fever for hot drinks; profuse sweat after fever;

great nervousness during paroxysms; intolerance of noise; irritable.

TISSUES

- Obstinate rheumatism.
- Sequelae of acute articular rheumatism; walks leaning on a cane, bent over; muffled in wraps to ears, looking like a broken down man apparently soon to ball into his grave.
- Glandular enlargement in various parts of body, with rachitis, in traced to hereditary gonorrhoea; patients are better at the seaside.

SKIN

- Copper coloured spots (syphilitic) remaining after eruptions, turn yellow brown & detach in scales, leaving skin charred & free.
- Itching < thinking of it.
- Trembling all over (subjective); intense nervousness & profound exhaustion.
- State of collapse, wants to be fanned all the time (*Carbo-v*); craves fresh air; skin cold, yet threw off the covers (*Camph., Sec.*); cold, & bathed with cold perspiration (*Verat.*)

Chapter 40

Syphilinum[3,4,17,21,34,39,48]

Secretion of syphilitic chancre

AUTHORITIES

Dr. Sam'l Swan, I.C. Boardman, Thomas Wider, E.A. Ballad Wm. Eggert, Laure Morgan, H.I. Ostrom, Wm. Bradshaw, Thomas Skinner, R.M. Theobald, S. Morrison, D.W. Clauson, C.F. Nichols, E.W. Berridge, Francis Buritt, S.W. Jackson, R.N. Foster, E.B. Nash, Julius Schmidt, C.W. Boyce, W.A. Howley, D.B. Morrow, J.R. Haynes, H.H. Carr, H.C. Allen, J.T. Kent.

HOW TO RECOGNIZE:

1. Syphilitic fear of disease.
2. Worse sundown to sunrise [Night].
3. Also present i) Punched out painless ulcer ii) Valvular Heart Disease iii) Aneurysm of Aorta.
4. Syphilitic gait = wide based, stamping gait.

5. Syphilitic mind: Paranoid destructive; Loss of memory; Loss of concentration Delusion of grandeur; Dementia; Insanity.
6. Syphilitic pain = Lightening, deep boring pain.
7. Face: disparity on side of face [Facial asymmetry] Unequal pupil, Sharp deformed teeth.
8. Obsessive compulsive.
9. Look older / Facial asymmetry / presence of stigma of congenital syphilis.
10. Congenital syphilis
    i) Failure to thrive [Marasmus etc.]
    ii) Anoxia/Hypoxia at birth
    iii) Peg teeth
    iv) Hepato–splenomegaly
    v) Neural involvement
    vi) Saddle nose
    vii) Interstitial keratitis
    viii) Tibial deformity

MENTALS

1. Fears many [Fear of night/illness/germs/insanity/financial ruin/robbers].
2. Fear of germs, hand–washing OCD.
3. Memory poor for names; recent events; & dates; concentration poor.
4. Paranoid(Persecution complex self–destructive, suicidal company aversion to, apathy alteration with irritability even violence.
5. Accident prone.

GENERALS

1. Aggravation
   Chilly yet < heat of bed
   < Night [Sunset to sunrise]
   < Sea side
   < Touch
   < Storm
   < Extremes of temperature
   < Heat of bed
2. Amelioration
   > Day
   > Mountain
   > Gentle motion [tub
   > Fast–motion]
3. Pain: Comes & goes slowly.
   : Deep boring pain / sharp stabbing pain.
   : Straight line pain.
4. Food: Aversion meat.

MATERIA MEDICA OF LUESINUM/ SYPHILINUM

MIND

- Cross, irritable, peevish.
- Very despondent, does not think that he will ever get better.

- Terrible dread of night, not on account of cough but on account of mental & physical exhaustion when she awakes; it is intolerable, death is preferable; she fears to prepare for night & is positively in object fear of suffering in form of exhaustion on awakening; it is < by cough, but it is quite independent of cough as she wakes in this awful state; always < as night approaches; leaves her about daylight, which she prays for.

HEAD

- Headache: linear, from or near one eye backward; lateral; frontal; from temple to temple; deep into brain from vertex; as from pressure on vertex; in either temple, extending into or from eye > by warmth; in bones of head; < by heat of sun; after sunstroke.
- Lancinating pain in occiput, < invariably at night, & causing sleeplessness, but always ceasing with the coming light of morning
- Neuralgic headache causing sleeplessness or delirium at night, always commencing about 4 p.m.; < at from 10 to 11 p.m., & ceasing at daylight.
- Headache through temples, then vertically like an inverted letter.
- Coronal headache.
- Headaches accompanied by great restlessness, sleeplessness & general nervous erethism.
- Syphilitic headache for many months, piercing, pressing excruciating over right eye; extending deep into brain; losing continuity of thought & memory; makes repeated mistakes in figures.
- Dirty eruption on scalp.

- Nervous chills preceded by aching pains in head, especially in occipital & integuments thereof, head feeling heavy, sore, congested; also frontal headache about one–half or two–thirds inches wide across forehead under eyebrows; aching pains below waist, in pelvis & extremities, especially in tibia, which is sensitive to touch; pains commence about 4 p.m., culminate about midnight in delirium, & cease entirely at day light.
- Syphilitic cephalgia in occiput, intolerable, extending to nervous ganglia of neck, causing hardness of cords, attacks at irregular intervals, especially after excitement.

EYES

- Red papulous eruption round left Inner canthus, with isolated pimples on side of nose, cheek & eyebrows; there pimples were red, with depressed center, circumscribed areola, became confluent where they were most dense; pimples bleed when scabs come off; agglutination of lids.
- Upper lid swollen.
- Ptosis: paralytic; eyes look sleepy from lowering of upper lid.
- Chronic recurrent phlyctenular inflammation of cornea; successive crops of phlyctenular and abrasion of epithelial layer of cornea; intense photophobia; profuse lachrymation; redness & pain well marked; delicate, scrofulous children, especially if any trace of hereditary syphilis remains.
- Left eyeball covered with fungus–like growth, pain intense < at night.
- Acute ophthalmia neonatorum.
- Redness & swelling of outer half of both lower tarsal edges.
- Syphilitic iritis, intense pain steadily increasing night after night; < between 2 & 5 a.m., coming almost at the minute & ceasing same way.

- Pain in rt. inner canthus as if blood went there & could go no further, also in rt. temple.
- Both eyes glued in morning; conjunctiva injected; photophobia, constantly wears a shade.
- Eyes dull.
- Ophthalmic pains, < at night, > by cold water.
- Right eye alone affected, congestion of conjunctiva & sclerotica, with some chemosis; lids inflamed, especially at outer canthus; sensation of sand in eyes; lids agglutinated in morning; great photophobia (hereditary syphilis).
- Neuralgia every night, beginning about 8 or 9 p.m., gradually increasing in severity until it reached its height about 3 or 4 A.M, and after continuing thus for two or three hours, gradually decreased & finally ceased about 10 a.m.; attacks gradually get more severe & last longer; first feel cold all over, almost a shiver; then soreness as if beaten in right half of head, extending a little beyond middle line on vertex; in about 30 min. scalding lachrymation from right eye, with shooting backward therein; eye is very red & closed, < photophobia; gnawing pains extending down right side of face & whole nose; head is worst when eye is bad; during paroxysms right feels as if lids were open wide, & cold air blowing on exposed eye; she perceives a horizontal band across pupil of right eye > by placing handkerchief on head & lifting it long over eyes, also by gentle pressure, though she cannot bear much pressure; it is more painful when lying on right (affected) side when also right side of head feels sore; right eye red, & red vessels run all over it. Right iris looks dull & there is a slight brown hue around pupil; left eye normal; attacks seem to have originated from sitting at a window in a cold draft.
- During sleep lids adhere; in infantile syphilis.

Syphilinum

- Paralysis of superior oblique.
- Chronic recurrent phlyctenular inflammation of cornea; successive crops of phlyctenular & abrasion of epithelial layer of cornea. Eyes very red & inflamed.
- Eyes swollen & cloud with syphilitic ophthalmia, pus running out of them.
- Pain in right inner canthus as if blood went there & could go no further, also in right temple.
- At 1 p.m. scalding lachrymation of rt. eye with shooting therein, followed by shooting from around eye into eye red & closed; this decreased & ceased about 3 p.m. recurred at same hour.
- On turning eye to left feels momentary coldness in inner half of right eye.
- On walking across room, right eye sensitive to air aches on using it. Left eye closed, up lid swollen as large as half an English walnut; deep red, not much pain, with oozing of purulent matter from between lids.

EARS

- Intense earache in right ear, incisive pains thrusting into ear; purulent watery discharge from ear with pain.
- Gathering in left ear which discharge a great quantity of pus (hereditary syphilis in a child).
- Deafness gradually increasing until she could scarcely hear at all.
- Complete deafness; nothing abnormal to seen.
- Catarrhal or nerve deafness with marked cachexia.
- Calcareous deposits on tympanum.
- Small, acrid, watery discharge occasionally from ears, no deafness (ozaena).

NOSE

- Attack of fluent coryza
- Offensive, thick yellow–green nasal discharges; during sleep dry scabs from in both nostrils; following an application of ointment for sore eyes; left submaxillary gland, with had been swollen & indurated, softens, discharges & after few days begins to heal slowly.
- Ozaena syphilitica. (*Syph*. Brought out on eruption of sores with a fiery–red base on nose over frontal sinuses)
- Left side of nose inside & out very sore, likewise lips & chin; sores itching & scabbing over; scabs falling off, leaving skin beneath of a dull–reddish copper colour.
- Itching in nostrils.

FACE

- Spasmodic twitching of many muscles, esp. in face (paralysis agitans), < great melancholy & depression of spirits.
- Facial paralysis right side thick speech, hemicrania.
- Face pale.
- Itching, scabby, eczematous eruption singly or in clusters looking like herpes.
- Nose & cheeks covered < eruptions & scabs in layers rising to a point.
- Dark purple lines between alae nasi & cheeks.
- Lips & teeth covered with bloody mucus.

TEETH MOUTH

- Felt like a worm in tooth, could not tell which tooth.

- Aphasia, difficulty of finding words; debility.
- Foetid breath.
- Tongue coated white, edges indented by teeth.
- Putrid taste in mouth before epileptic fit.
- Tongue very red & thick; covered with herpetic eruption two deep cracks running lengthwise on each side of median line, making it difficult to swallow.
- Herpetic eruption in mouth, tonsils, hard palate & fauces, completely covering inside of mouth & throat, making it difficult to swallow even liquids.

THROAT

- Chronic hypertrophy of tonsil.
- Chancrous ulcers extending across velum palate to lt. pillar of pharynx, which was thickened, interfering very much with his speech; voice husky.
- Acute pharyngitis.

APPETITE

- Appetite indifferent & capricious.
- Total loss of appetite for months, little or nothing satisfies him, formerly was generally ravenous.
- Lose of appetite.
- Tendency to heavy drinking; alcoholism.
- Aversion to meat.
- Dyspepsia; flatulence, belching of wind; nervous dyspepsia.

STOMACH

- Heartburn with pain & rawness from stomach to throat pit, after with cough.
- Vomiting for weeks or months due to erosion from superficial ulceration of lining of viscus herpetic of syphilitic origin.

ABDOMEN

- Large painless bubo in rt. groin opened & discharged freely.
- Inguinal bubo.

STOOL & ANUS

- Obstinate constipation for many years; rectum seemed tied up with strictures when injections were given agony of passage was like child–bearing.
- Bowels sluggish for five weeks.
- Stools very dark & offensive.
- Stools too light coloured.
- Bilious diarrhoea at seashore, painless, driving her out of bed about 5 a.m.; stools during day; later causing excoriation; face red, suffers from heat; occasional painless, whitish diarrhoea when at cholera, > always by going to mountains.
- Obstinate cases of cholera infantum.
- Fissures in anus & rectum.
- Indurated ulcers at mouth of anus somewhat sore; slight itching of anus.
- Lower portion of rectum hanging out like a ruffle, looking like a full–blown rose fully 3 inches in diameter, sensitive; constant weak dragging sensation in rectum, extending as for as sacrum.

URINARY ORGANS

- Urination difficult & very slow; no pain, but a want of power, so that he has to strain.
- Urine infrequent, not oftener than once in 24 hr.; scanty, of a golden–yellow colour.
- Profuse urination after chill; passed during night nearly a chamberful.
- Rich lemon–yellow scanty urine.
- Frequent urging to urinate all night, at least from 7 p.m. until 5 a.m. sunset to sunrise.

MALE

- Chancre on prepuce.
- Buboes.
- Chancre on penis, third in two years, all on same spot.
- After suppressed chancre, disease attacked testes & scrotum, which become painful & swollen; this was supposed to be cured, but ever since, every few weeks, if exposed to damp weather would be seized with pain as if in kidneys, seemingly traversing ureters, but instead of passing into bladder followed spermatic cord, down groins & into testes; pain agonizing, chiefly in cord; pricking in chancre, as though punctured by pins.
- Chancroid, Phagedenic, spreading rapidly; buboes commencing in each groin.
- Inflammation & induration of spermatic cord.
- Constant pain in anterior Part of leg. Thigh < while standing painful all night, preventing sleep; bubo in lt. inguinal region size of pigeons egg, purple, fluctuating; night sweats.

FEMALE

- Uterine & all surrounding parts loose, soft & flabby; profuse, thick, yellow leucorrhoea; constant pain across small of back.
- Yellow offensive leucorrhoea, watery or not, so profuse it daily soaks through napkin & runs to heels of stocking if much on her feet.
- Profuse yellow leucorrhoea < at night; in sickly, nervous children.
- Soreness of genitals, & muco–purulent discharge, in a child.
- Acrid discharge causing violent itching & inflammation of external organs < at night from warmth of bed, parts very tender; itching & inflammation > during menses.
- Nocturnal < of right ovarian pain, preventing sleep.
- Sore spot on right labium majus, extending to left.
- Painful menstruation.
- Ovaries congested & inflamed; tendency to ovarian tumors.
- Uterine & ovarian diseases < pronounced nervous disorders, esp. in married women.

RESPIRATORY ORGANS

- Diseased cartilages of larynx.
- Attacks of spasmodic bronchial asthma, they come on only at night after lying down or during a thunder–storm, producing most intense nervous insomnia, entirely preventing sleep for days & nights.
- Violent attacks of dyspnoea, wheezing & rattling of mucus, from 1 to 4 a.m.

COUGH

- Dry, racking cough, with thick, purulent expectoration, caused by a sensation of rasping or scraping in throat, always < at night.
- Whooping cough < terrible vomiting.
- Cannot lie on right side as it causes a dry cough.
- Muco–purulent expectoration, greyish, greenish, greenish–yellow tasteless.
- Expectoration without cough, quite clear, white, feels like a round ball & rushes into mouth.
- Dry, short, hacking cough without expectoration, but < rawness, scrapping & burning from faces to stomach pit; with a whooping in inspiration & a choking sensation from faces to bifurcation of bronchia, great mental distress.

CHEST

- Chronic asthma; in summer, esp. when weather was warm & damp; most frequently in evening; soreness of chest, < great anguish & inability to retain a recumbent position; in winter severe bronchial cough succeeded by asthmatic attacks; a regular type of chills & fever developed.
- Rattling in chest & throat.
- Pain & pressure behind sternum.
- Angina; ptosis left eye; facial paralysis left side, slight aphasia; impotence.
- Eczematous herpetic eruptions on chest.
- Asthma only at night after lying sown, or during a thunderstorm.

NECK & BACK

- Heavy aching & stiffness from base of neck up through muscles & cards into brain.
- Great pain in back in region of kidneys, < after urinating.
- Caries of cervical spine with great curvature in same region, directly forward, occiput sinking down to a level with it & resting on protuberance of curvature; calcareous matter would be discharged & on evaporating it a quantity of dry powder, looking like phosphate of lime, would be felt; pain in curvature always < at night (no proof of syphilis).
- Caries or dorsal vertebrae < acute curvature.
- Enlargement of cervical glands & a number of pedunculated pin head warts on neck; cured by syco–syphilinum.
- Nocturnal aggravation of pains in back, hips & thighs.
- Enormous swelling of glands in head & neck.

UPPER LIMB

- Rheumatism of shoulder joint or at insertion of deltoid, < from raising arm laterally.
- Fingers & thumbs have run around (infantile syphilis).
- Hands badly ulcerated on backs.
- Right second finger is swollen backs.

LOWER LIMB

- Every winter intense cold pain in both legs, < in left came on every night or lying down, lasting all night; > by setting up & walking, & in warm weather.
- Slight contraction of tendons beneath right knee.

- Redness & rawness with terrible itching between toes.
- Bubo with pain in spot in spot in spot on middle of thigh in front, only, which was apparently on periosteum.
- Large ulcers, dirty sinking, sloughing, < jagged, elevated edges, over the bony surface, from which large pieces of bone come away.
- Osteosarcoma in centre of right tibia the size of half an ostrich egg, pains agonizing at night, growth irregular, spongy, partly laminated, very hard.
- Contracted, painful feeling in soles, as if tendons were too short.
- Rheumatic swelling of wrist & big toe, bluish red, < pains as if somebody sawed at his bones will a bull sow; > by heat of stove; < from sundown to sunrise.
- Excruciating arthritis; swelling, heat, & redness intense.
- Severe attack of aching in lower limbs.
- Sharp rheumatic pain, burning like fire, in instep & below inner malleolus, prevents moving foot < when toe is pointed inward; <in evening, continuing during night, < toward day break.

SKIN

- Bitting sensation in different parts of body, as if bitten by bugs, at night only.
- Syphilitic rash an abundance on forehead, chin arms & front of thorax, an abundance of fine scaly peeling off large prominent spot on centre of forehead, filled with fluid as also are some smaller patches.
- Syphilitc bulla discharging freely on cheeks, under chin, on back of shoulders, on scalp & other parts of body (infantile syphilis).
- Macula; copper coloured; from crown of head to sole of foot.

- Pemphigus, looking like a pock, often confluent & persistently reappears. Skin bluish.
- Macula over back, chest, abdomen, arms & legs, but not on any uncovered part of body.
- Several elevated spots on arms, stomach, legs & finger; has them habitually on face, chiefly on lt. cheek.
- A blood boil on arm' face broken out with a lumpy fiery rash.
- Eruption over whole body not elevated, but could be distinctly felt by passing hand over skin; after syphilinum 1M. Eruption came rapidly to surface, disagreeable odour began to be developed, eruption reddish – brown like small–pox pustules, without central depression; body covered < it; completely covering inside of mouth & throat; eyes also closed; intolerable smell from body; tips of pimples become filled < pus; < from warmth of bed; foetid breath; eruption developed still more, a great quantity of pus, < intolerable itching, yet could not scratch as it was extremely sore; eruption left skin of entire body covered with dull, reddish, copper coloured spots, which in cold, looked blue.

SLEEP

- Absolute sleeplessness. (vies with sulph in producing quiet, refreshing sleep).

FEVER

- Great Pains in head, whole body extremely cold, looked blue; wanted to be covered with blankets or couldn't get warm; no appetite; sleeping almost continually, could not be aroused.
- Nervous chills preceded by pains in head, esp. occiput & scalp of that part; pains below waist, in pelvis, legs, esp. tibia, which is sensitive to touch; bowels torpid; cross, irritable, peevish; pains

Syphilinum

- begin every day at 4 p.m., culminate at midnight, disappear at daylight.
- Sweat; profuse at night, sleepless & restless; esp. between scapulae & down to waist, with excessive general debility.
- Fever from 11 to 1 p.m. daily; perspires when she begins to get over fever; pain in back, < between shoulders, no ambition or desire to move.
- Excessive general debility & continued night sweat latter being most marked between scapulae & down to waist.

HOW & WHEN TO USE LEUSINUM:

1. Pains from darkness to daylight; begins with twilight & ends with daylight. (*Merc, Phyt.*).
2. Pains increases & decreases gradually (*Stann.*); shifting & require frequent change of position.
3. All symptoms are worse at night (*Merc*).
4. Eruption: dull, red, copper coloured spots, becoming blue when getting cold.
5. Extreme emaciation of entire body (Abrot, Iod) – Heart: lancinating pains from base to apex, at night (from apex to base – Med); from base to clavicle, or shoulder (*Spig.*).
6. Loss of memory: cannot remember names of books, persons or places; arithmetical calculations difficult.
7. Sensations: as if going insane: if about to be paralyzed; of apathy & indifference.
8. Terrible dread of night on account of mental & physical exhaustion on awakening; it is intolerable, death is preferable.
9. Fears the terrible suffering from exhaustion on awakening (*Lach*).

10. Leucorrhoea: profuse, soaking through the napkins & running down to heels (Alum)
11. Headache, neuralgic in character, causing sleeplessness & delirium at night; commencing at 4 p.m.; worse from 10 to 11 & ceasing at daylight (ceases at 11 or 12 p.m. – *Lyc.*); falling of hairs.
12. Ophthalmia neonatorum; lids swollen, adhere during sleep; pain intense at night < from 2–5 a.m.; pus profuse; > cold bathing.
13. Ptosis: paralysis of superior oblique; sleepy look from drooping lids (*Caust, Graph.*)
14. Diplopia, one image seen below the other.
15. Teeth: decay at edge of gum & break off; are cupped, edges serrated; dwarfed in size, converge at their tips (*Staph*).
16. Craving alcohol in any form. Hereditary tendency to alcoholism (*Sars, Psor., Tuber, Sulph., Sulph-ac*)
17. Obstinate constipation for years; rectum seems tied up with strictures; when enemata were used the agony of passage was like labour (*Lac-d., Tub.*)
18. Fissures in anus & rectum (*Thuja*); Prolapse of rectum; obstinate case with a syphilitic history.
19. Rheumatism of the shoulder joint, or at insertion of deltoid, < from raising arm laterally (*Rhus*, right shoulder – *Sang*; left – *Ferr.*)
20. When the best selected remedy fails to relieve or permanently improve in syphilitic affections.
21. Syphilitics, or patients Who have had chancre treated by local means, and as a result have suffered from throat & skin troubles for years, are nearly always benefited by this remedy at commencement of treatment unless some other remedy is clearly indicated.

RELATIONS

- Antidote; *Nux-v.*, for over–action or excess of action in sensitive organizations, or too frequent repetition of the remedy, especially in the higher potencies.

COMPARE

- *Aur, Asaf, Kali–iod, Mer., Phyr., Nit–ac* in diseases of bone & syphilitic affections.
- *Ech., Lac–can., Med.,* in dysmenorrhoea.
- *Calc., Tub.,* headache deep in the brain.
- *Plat., Stan.,* Pains increase & decrease slowly.
- *Alum., Kali-bi., Puls., Psor., Sep., Teuc.,* Post nasal catarrh, or ozena, with offensive plugs or clinkers.
- *Hep. Sulph, Sil, Psor.,* tendency to successive abscesses (succession of boils Anthr.,).
- *Aur., Lac. Can., Lach., Mer-i.,* Syphiltic stomatitis.
- *Calc. Flour-ac., Kali-bi., Kali-i., Mang., Merc.,* Syphilitic nodes.
- *Abrot, Iod., Tub.,* Progressive emaciation.
- *Med.,* lancinating pain in heart (from apex to Base). *Spig.* (from base to clavicle or shoulder) *Syph.* (from Base to apex).
- *Lach.,* fear of Exhaustion on awakening.
- *Caust., Gels., Graph.,* Paralysis of up. Lids.
- *Asar., Med., Psor., Sull., Tub.,* hereditary tendency to alcoholism.
- *Lac., Tub.,* Paralytic weakness of rectum with labour like pains.
- *Nat-m., Sanic., Thuja,* fissure ani.
- *Kreos., Merc.,* troubles during dentition, especially if hereditary syphilis be suspected.
- *Phos., X–ray,* bad effects of thunder–storms.

Chapter 41

Tuberculinum [3,4,10,19,21,23,31,34,39,41,47,48]

MATERIA MEDICA OF TUBERCULINUM

MIND

- Irritable on talking; nothing can please him, nothing satisfies.
- With every little ailment whines & complains; easily frightened, particularly dogs; screams in terror when approached by a dogs.
- Although naturally of a sweet disposition, become taciturn sulky, snappish, fretty, irritable, morose, depressed & melancholic, even to insanity – Burnett

HEAD

- Severe headache, < on second day, lasting until the third, recurring from time to time for many weeks & compelling quiet fixedness – Burnett
- Headache, < frequent sharp, cutting pains passing from above right eye. Through head to back of left ear – Rose

- Headache of great intensity preceded by a shuddering chill passing from brain down spine, with attack a feeling as if head above eyes were swollen; become unconscious with screaming, tearing her hair, beating her head with her fists or trying to dash it against wall or floor – Swan
- Headache of 45 yrs. standing, pain passing from right frontal protuberance to right occipital region– Swan
- Terrible pain in head, as if he had a tight hoop of iron around it; trembling of hands; distressing sensation of damp clothes on his spine; almost absolute sleeplessness; profound adynamia; was thought by his friends to be on verge of insanity; most of his brothers & sisters had died of water on brain; right lung solid, probably from healed up cavities, as he at one time suffered from pulmonary phthisis – Burnett
- Sullen, taciturn, irritable, screams in his sleep, is very restless at night, constipated; sister died of tubercular meningitis – Burnett
- Fretful & ailing, whines & complains, indurated glands can be felt every where, child hot, drowsy, urine red & sandy, must given to be frightened, Particularly by dogs; was vaccinated & had a very bad arm for four months thereafter; would not smile, whimpers when spoken to, skin dingy, skull, hydrocephalic – Burnett
- Boy, aged 20 months, ill for days < head, high fever, restlessness & constant screaming; finally no sleep for forty hours, followed by a condition of collapse, peculiar smell of body, family history of T.B. – Burnett
- Tubercular meningitis, < effusion; head gradually enlarged; alternately wakeful & delirious at night., talked nothing by day, at intervals; nocturnal hallucinations & fright, delirium; pyrexia; had eczema which almost disappeared after two unsuccessful vaccinations, & which were soon followed by above condition;

after administration of remedy there occurred a severe pustular eruption, then patches of a lepra & eczema appeared.
- Basilar meningitis – Sinker
- Tubercular meningitis – Sinker
- Acute cerebral meningitis, < intense strabismus – Biegler
- Plica polonica; several bad cases permanently cured with *Tub.* – Jackson

NOSE

- Soreness inside of nose, commencing as watery pimples, which, suppurating, from scabs; nose & lips somewhat swollen; itching slightly – Rose

FACE

- Slight swelling & itching of lips – Rose

STOMACH

- Windy dyspepsia, < pinching & pains under rids of right side in mammary line – Burnett

ABDOMEN

- Fever, emaciation, abdominal pains & discomfort, restlessness at right, glands of both groins enlarged & indurated; cries out in sleep; strawberry tongue – Burnett
- Tabes mesenterica; swelling on left side, also on right; complains of a stitch in side after running; languid & indisposed to talk; nervous & irritable; talks in his sleep; grinds his teeth; appetite poor; hands blue; indurated & palpable glands every where; a drum belly; spleen region bulging out – Burnett

- Inguinal glands indurated & visible; excessive sweats; chronic diarrhoea.

STOOL ANUS

- Diarrhoea, furious fever, burning hot skin, great heat in head, red, flushed face, eyes turned upward, quivering & rolling; peculiar foetid smell of body – Burnett.
- Cholera infantum – Swan.
- Severe haemorrhage from bowels, cough; emaciation; family history of phthisis.

RESPIRATORY ORGANS

- Expectoration diminished – Heron (H.C. Allen).
- Copious watery expectoration usually seen during the reaction – Wilson.
- Extreme rapidity of respirations, without dyspnoea, 60 to 90 per minute; if the patient is spoken to, the rapid breathing ceases at once (as with a dog panting in the sun). – Heron (H.C. Allen).
- Slight tedious hacking cough, which had lasted for months in a girl of a distinctly phthisic habit – Burnett.
- Hard, dry cough, sometimes slight, but generally no expectoration, slightly feverish – Boardman (H.C. Allen).
- Expectoration of non – viscid, very easily detached, thick phlegm from air passages, followed after a day or two by a very clear ring of voice – Burnett.

CHEST

- Slight hacking cough, continuing all day, < at bedtime & on rising; emaciation; dullness on percussions at apex of right lung – Burnett.

- Girl, aged 15, tall; tonsils enlarged; chronic discharge from nose, < early morning on rising; speech thick; thorax of pigeon–breast type; perspires much across nose; very bad perspiration of chest, armpits, palms, & feet; feels very chilly; spleen swollen; district dullness on percussion at apex of right lung; suffered badly from vaccination; gets chilblains – Burnett.

- Hectic flush of cheeks; shortness of breath; slight hacking cough; several strumous scars on neck; dusky skin; large, moist rales in both lungs; increased vocal resonance of right lung; amphoric sounds in right lung; large soft feeling glands in left side of neck; very pronounced endocardial bruit best heard at apex beat. *Iodoformicum* 3X in four grain dose for two months, < improvement, followed by *Tuberculinum* in very infrequent doses – Burnett.

- Incipient phthisis in a boy aged 7; lass of flesh; great prostration; morbid timidity; glands of groins, on both side of neck very much enlarged & indurated, particularly glands over apex of right lung; as he had suffered much from vaccination. *Thuja* 30 & *Sabina* 30 were first used then *Tuberculinum* – Burnett.

- Nocturnal perspiration; notched incisors; indurated glands everywhere, very large & numerous; drum bellied; grinding of teeth at rt; great susceptibility to taking cold; perspiration < at back of lungs & on head; big head,< bulging forehead; subject to attacks of fever & diarrhoea – Burnett.

- Incipient tubercular disease Restless at night.; sleepless; grinds teeth; tendency to diarrhoea; want of appetite; frail breath; notched teeth; pain after food; vomiting of food; indurated glands; strawberry tongue; naughty; very irritable temper; puny growth; very thin, girl, aged 6 – Burnett.

- A nasty little cough; for seven weeks; much expectoration, pain in rt. lung; evening fever; liver & spleen enlarged; cough morning after breakfast; neck slightly goitrous; eats hardly any breakfast – Burnett.

– Cough, < 6 a.m.; notched incisors, thin & puny; cervical & inguinal glands much enlarged & indurated; strawberry tongue; girl, aged 7 – Burnett.

– No respiratory sounds at top of right Lung, vocal resonance slightly increased; pain in left side; profuse perspiration; girl, aged 18 – Burnett.

– Much fever, < evenings; restless & terribly irritable; much depressed & in almost constant agitation; tongue very red; chronic diarrhoea; has lost fourteen pounds during last six weeks; has no appetite; evacuation discharged from bowels as from a pop–gun – Burnett.

– Bad cough of about twelve month's duration; expectoration of blood; one of apices was audibly diseased; has had pneumonia; chest flat; respiration accelerated; tanned unduly in sun – Burnett.

– Anaemic, sickly, pale; profound debility; dysponea, can't mount or hurry; menses irregular – Burnett.

– Lady, aged 26, in first stage of consumption, dysponea & rapid breathing; loss of flesh; greasy, dingy skin – Burnett.

– Stout man, bright, florid complexion, mother died of phthisis; gets pneumonia very after in cold weather; hence travels from place to place to avoid colds; cough much, brings up much fluids; wretched sleepless nights, < almost constant fever; glands of neck much enlarged – Burnett.

– Complains that she has been in consumption for many years; is very thin and consumed < fever; lungs very flat; respiration almost imperceptible; fever; poor appetite; languid – Burnett.

– Ringworm on scalp; lymphatic glands everywhere palpable; ribs very flat; strawberry tongue, bad cough, < at night although 11

- years old she had practically no teeth, they were rudimentary, & not above level of gums – Burnett.
- Pronounced phthisical habit; severe piles; constipation; brown cutaneous affection on abdomen – Burnett.
- I always hesitate to gives the remedy first hand, but have a number of times and it after other remedies failed, & with success, especially where there was a tubercular tendency – Scholes.

HEART

- Death from paralysis of heart – Libherts.

NECK & BACK

- Violent reaction, during which pain in loins < by pressure; (Case of Addisons disease) – Pick.
- Tuberculosis of sacrum greatly improved – Kurz.
- Indurated cervical glands.
- Lump, size of a walnut on cord of neck, is movable & occasionally itches – Rose.

LOWER LIMB

- Swelling & tenderness of both knee joints – Heron (H.C. Allen)
- Tubercular swelling of knee; intermittent attacks of pain in it; has expectorated clots of blood & suffered from exhausting sweats; family history of phthisis – Burnett.
- Tuberculous disease of left knee, for eleven months had been limping; Knee much enlarged & very tender; teeth dirty & carious; strawberry tongue – Burnett.

SKIN

- Very bad tempered; very much pigmented where suns rays impinged upon him; teeth dirty, greenish – Burnett.
- Ringworm.

SLEEP

- Disturbed distressful sleep – Burnett.

FEVER

- Feverish, nausea, thirsty, < headache, no vomiting – Heron (H.C. Allen).
- Lowering of temperature after each injection – Heron (H.C. Allen).
- Lowering of temperature after a rise – Heron (H.C. Allen).
- Temperature seven hours after injection, 103.8° accompanied by thirst, rigor, increased cough, headache, and pains in joints – Heron (H.C. Allen).

NERVES

- Suddenly become unconscious while sewing or talking, began screaming, tearing her hair, beating her head with her fists or trying to dash it against the wall or floor; attacks daily for a month, then spasms set in < rolling of head from side to side & moaning; continuing 5 weeks, followed by a recurrence of fainting fits, at least twice a weeks; a few hour before an attack of fainting a shuddering like a chill seemed to go from brain down spine when questioned about an attack, she said head would suddenly seem to swell over eyes & pain becomes "horrid" & she knew no more; between attacks she was free from all complaints except fatigue & an ever-present frontal headache – Swan.

GENERALITIES

- Oxyhaemoglobin first diminished then increased – Henoque.
- Where tubercle is associated with any other specific disease, reaction is so slight as to be scarcely discernible – Heron (H.C. Allen).
- Syphilitic cases are refractory to reaction – (H.C. Allen).
- Children bear the treatment well – Wendt.

Chapter 42

Carcinosin [14,19,32,38,39,45]

With the incidence of cancer rising, it is no surprise that the prescriptions for *Carcinosin* are increasing too. Whether the judicious use of *Carcinosin* will reduce the future number of cancers remains to be seen. Thanks to the work of Donald Foubister and those that followed in his footsteps, a coherent picture of the *Carcinosin* personality has emerged from provings and sound clinical experience. It is extremely close to the Type C / Cancer personality described by psychologists.

There is now firm evidence that the psychological profile of a person affects their susceptibility to disease. Psycho-Neuroimmunology provides the mechanism behind the inter-play of emotions and physical disease. There are many ways in which the resilience of an individual may be increased in the face of a disadvantage start to life as in the *Carcinosin* scenario.

No longer can "conventional" Medicine ignore the fundamental unity of mind, body and soul. To quote George Vithoulkas *"disease is the discipline of the human being in its upward march for spiritual evolution"*.

Carcinosin is a very deep acting remedy which brings about profound changes in our patients on every level of their existence.

David Lilley says that cancer is the "ultimate healing". With such a wonderful remedy as *Carcinosin*, healing can begin prior to the manifestation of physical dis-ease.

HISTORY OF CARCINOSIN

Carcinosin was first introduced as a palliative remedy for the treatment of malignancy by Kent, Compton Burnett and J.H. Clarke also used the remedy. In addition to palliative uses, they noticed the miasmatic traits and psychological components albeit in a primitive rudimentary form. Boericke added rheumatism, abdominal bloating and indigestion to the potential uses.

The major contribution to the evolution of the Materia Medica of *Carcinosin* was by Donald Foubister in the 1950's. The proving done by Templeton and Hui Bon Hoa added further valuable information.

Foubister's interest in the remedy was ignited when he saw two children born to mothers with breast cancer and was struck by the similarities in their appearance - the blue-sclerotics, cafe au lait spots and multiple moles - and their presenting symptom, insomnia. Using astute clinical observation and meticulous records of over 200 Cancer cases, in his Paediatric clinics, he published "Clinical Impressions of *Carcinosin*". in the British homoeopathic Journal in 1954.

Already in this paper are very clear instructions of the mental state of the remedy. The suppression of emotions, prolonged fear and unhappiness, anticipatory anxiety, intense sympathy empathy, the inability to stand up for oneself, fastidiousness, emotional insecurity, sensitivity to reprimand, aversion to consolation and the gentle disposition of the "good" child are well described. Interestingly, the mental symptoms of one child are under-emphasised, because of "the shock and grief of her mother's death from cancer".

The frame-work of all the physical symptoms that are associated with cancer miasm is also evident. Foubister also noted the strong family history of other diathetic conditions. Despite Kent's assertion that cancer was the result of suppressed psora, it is now generally believed in homoeopathic circles, that it is a multi-miasmatic condition, as suggested by Paterson.

Later Foubister, supplied with operation samples from the Royal London Homoeopathic Hospital, produced a selection of remedies from various tumours. He found these far more potent than the original and advised they be used with caution. These newer *Carcinosin* have never been formally proved and probably do represent a slightly different drug picture. In his book "Tutorials in Homoeopathy" Foubister demonstrates a few keynotes of the remedies. With Foubister's assertion that this was a constitutional remedy as well as a nosode, more homoeopath's began to use the remedy and other indications for its use came to light. Paschero in Argentina found *Carcinosin* reduced the incidence of keloid scars after plastic surgery and Shapiro added it to the list of remedies for the ill effects of vaccination.

Over the years there have been a lot of valuable contributions to the understanding of *Carcinosin*, which elaborate on the basic picture as resented by Foubister.

THE REMEDY PICTURE OF CARCINOSIN

It is essential that homoeopaths have a good understanding of the remedy picture of *Carcinosin* in order to make use of such valuable remedy.

As the incidence of cancer increases, there is great potential for its use. Homoeopaths may be divided into two groups as to the place of the remedy in cancer and this can be traced back to Kent's comment on its use in palliative treatment. Foubister held a contrary opinion stating that "the further away you get from the actual cancer, as in childhood, more useful *Carcinosin* is as a constitutional remedy". He also states that "it is not without danger to give *Carcinosin* to cancer suspects".

THE INHERITANCE OF CARCINOSIN

According to Foubister, the *Carcinosin* child is often born into a family with a higher than average incidence of serious illness, such as tuberculosis, diabetes mellitus, pernicious anaemia and cancer.

The combination of three classic Hahnemannian miasms, psora, sycosis and syphilis, plus the tubercular diathesis (syco-syphilitic) produce the *Carcinosin* miasm.

A genetic predisposition for cancer is well recognised, for example in breast and colonic cancer (familial polyposis coli.) However, not all members of the family express the cancer so other factors must be at play. Phenotype results from the interplay between genotype and the environment. Foubister noted that cancer has more common on the material side of the family.

THE GRIEF OF CARCINOSIN

Early grief and the subsequent disruption of the family unit affects "the development of personality, coping ability and social competence. The same is true of pronounced martial discord and the lack of adequate parental emotion affiliation and stimulation". These stresses have implications on the immune system, which will be discussed later.

In view of the family history, it is not surprising to find *Carcinosin* listed under ailments from grief.

CARCINOSIN AND TOO MUCH PARENTAL CONTROL

Carcinosin features under the rubrics for ailments from abuse, yet there is little mention of this until recently in the literature. Clarke noted that it was useful in treating "conditions in the children, such as infantile self-abuse." This closely echoes the prolonged fear and unhappiness quoted by Foubister although he does not mention a specific cause.

PSYCHOLOGICAL CONSEQUENCES OF PARENTAL CONTROL

According to Milton Erickson, a betrayal of trust can lead to hopelessness, a sense of lack of self worth, fear of being alone or of abandonment, and a lack of emotional boundaries. In addition there is the associated guilt, that may lead to a sense of over-responsibility for others and self loathing. All of these characteristics have been described in the *Carcinosin* personality.

Emotional and verbal abuse has destructive effect on the child's developing character and these experiences may lead to characteristic behavioural patterns. Tinus Smits explains the role of the father figure in the child's development. "The father is the symbol of self confidence, of strength, of social position and the realisation of the possibilities of the child." Domination, harsh upbringing and excessive parental control are all potentially damaging to the child.

In an attempt to avoid criticism, the child may behave impeccably, be "too well behaved", suppressing their natural spirit, their "inner child".

Many *Carcinosin* children grow up believing that their parent's love is conditional on good behaviour and academic achievements. This may lead to performance anxiety and perfectionist tendencies in later life. Over-anxious or overprotective parents may also stunt their child's development. The constant striving for perfection is considered by many authors to be a classic trait amongst those requiring *Carcinosin*, as a need for control in their life.

Brian Kaplan describes the essence of *Carcinosin* as "chaos" In order to combat this feeling, fastidiousness and perfectionist traits may occur. External order is a form of compensation for the internal chaos. This behaviour may develop into full blown obsessive compulsive disorder.

CARCINOSIN AND EARLY CHILDHOOD

Physically lacking in strength, and with further stressing of the immune system, there may be a history of pneumonia and whooping cough in young children and abnormal reactions to childhood infections. Intellectually, the *Carcinosin* child may be lacking (e.g. Down's syndrome) or very intelligent. *Carcinosin* is a remedy of contradiction, possibly as an expression of the underlying sycotic taint, hence there can be dyslexia or an excessive desire to read or a mixture of both. Losing oneself in a book is a form of escapism, as are computer games and television. These pursuits provide an escape from the deep emotional pain that some of these children experience. Dancing also provides an outlet. Art also provides a sanctuary of inner peace, and it opens up the "right brain". *Carcinosin* types are very creative.

CARCINOSIN AND ADOLESCENTS

As the child matures and enters puberty, the identity begins to evolve, a sense of self emerges. Teenage rebelliousness may be excessive in *Carcinosin*.

Eating disorders may develop as a need for control. Addiction to alcohol, drugs (including tobacco) or sex can also be seen. Sex, drugs and alcohol numb the mind and later consciousness. Food and sex can be replacements for the unconditional love these people seek so desperately and that has been denied them. Chaim Rosenthal sees drug addiction as the ultimate manifestation of the cancer miasm.

CARCINOSIN AND PERSONAL BOUNDARIES

In the *Carcinosin* personality, there is blurring of the personal boundaries. This leads to a high incidence of co-dependent relationships. There is an empathy for others to an unhealthy degree, tragic events affect them profoundly, possibly as a consequence of the resonance with their own suffering. *Carcinosin* patients literally feel the pain of others.

The lack of personal boundaries might be the explanation for the abnormal sensitivity to medication, acupuncture (strong reactors), hypnosis (mesmerism) and also environmental pollutants.

CARCINOSIN AND SEXUAL HEALTH

Carcinosin is useful in treating many gynaecological conditions; endometriosis, menstrual disturbances, and polycystic ovarian syndrome and disease. It has a great effect on regulating hormones, whether pituitary, adrenal, thyroid, pancreatic or sexual.

Typology / Constitution Carbonic & Phosphoric, Café-au-Lait Spots, Blue Sclerotics, Moles, Pale Complexion, Tubercular Physique, Sleeps in genupectoral position.

ESSENTIAL FEATURES FOR THE PRESCRIPTION OF CARCINOSIN

Dr. Foubister gives the following indications for the prescription of *Carcinosin*:

- A family history of a tendency to Cancer, Diabetes, Tuberculosis, Pernicious Anemia or a combination of these.
- A personal history of Whooping Cough or other severe acute infection at an early age.
- Marked aggravation / amelioration at the seaside.

WHEN TO THINK OF CARCINOSIN

1. Essence match.
2. When well selected remedy fails and cancer miasma can be observed.
3. The patient is partly covered by two or more of constitutional remedies, or when apparently clearly indicated related remedies do not work or have a very short action.

DRUG RELATIONSHIP

1. AVOIDING criticism, earnest, responsible, timid approach to life, Avoiding Conflicts, Reserved, Create Fantasy World, Loves Music & Dance, Weeps Listening to Music, Dreams of Harmony & Peace: *Thuja, Nat-m., Nat-c, Aur, Calc., Mang., Con.*
2. Becoming brilliant, ill at ease with people as good as him, Arrogant, Critical of others, Need Admiration *Lyco., Verat.,*

Sil., Caust., Staph., Puls., Phos., Sulph., Alum.

3. Conscientious, Fastidious, Control freaks, Persevering, Well Organised, Leaves nothing to chance (but are untidy at home), Anticipatory anxiety, Fear narrow place, Fear high place: *Ars., Nux-v., Med., Lyc., Puls., Sulph, Nat-m.*

4. Denial/avoidance, Easily offended, Sensitive to Reprimands, Obstinate, Incapable of admitting their mistakes, Afraid to perform to avoid disappointment, Refusal to do a job because of fundamental lack of confidence: *Puls., Staph., Sep., Plat., Pall., Cupr.*

IS CARCINOSIN INDICATED IN CASES OF CANCER

Dr. Foubister writes: in the homoeopathic recorder: "it must be that it is not without danger to give *Carcinosin* to cancer subjects". It has often been used in the treatment of cancer. Although it is claimed to relieve the pain of breast cancer but there are no records of cases of cancer treated by *Carcinosin* alone, and it is doubtful whether it is of much value in the disease. " It seems that the further away you are from cancer, the more valuable it is as a constitutional remedy".

Kent, comments in lesser writing:" *Carcinosin* relives pain that is sharp, burning or tearing with this remedy patients remained comfortable for many years, even though cure was impossible and the cancer continued to develop. The growth of the tumor was delayed and the suffering, which usually goes with this condition was avoided. This preparation is used with good effect in many cases of advanced epithelioma".

DIFFERENT CARCINOCIN PREPARATIONS

1. *Carcinoma*   : [Kent]
2. *Carcinosin*   : [Foubister]
3. *Schirrinum*   : [Burnett]
4. Newer *Carcinosin* : [Nelsons]
5. Mixed *Carcinosin*
   - C – Nosode Mix [Smits]
   - *Carcinosin* Co. [Nelsons]

MATERIA MEDICA OF CARCINOSIN

MIND

1. Absent – Minded.
2. Affectionate.
3. Ailments from; Anticipation; Fear; Fright, reproaches; rudeness of others; from a Long history of domination or excessive parental control; prolonged unhappiness, due to other people influence (e.g. a prolonged fear in a Child from domination by a Sadistic father).
4. Anger; over his mistake.
5. Anticipation; before examination.
6. Anxiety; about his Family, about others, because he is protected by the family. He has not the same protection in the Company of other People.
7. Bite; bites fingers.
8. Caresses; Propensity for Caresses.

9. Cheerful; gay, mirthful, cheerful when it Thunders and at Lightnings.
10. Clairvoyance
11. Not easily Satisfied.
12. Fear of Failure.
13. Concentration is difficult; difficult Concentration in Children.
14. Confusion of mind.
15. Conscientious; about trifles.
16. Consolations; aggravates or Kind words aggravates.
17. Contradiction is intolerant of.
18. Conversation aggravates; aversion to Conversion.
19. Dancing; Love of dancing; desire to dance
20. Delusions, as if arms do not belong to her.
21. Discontented; displeased, dissatisfied.
22. Domination; or excessive parental Control long history of domination.
23. Duty; excessive Sense of duty.
24. Dullness; Sluggishness in Children.
25. Fastidious;
26. Fear; apprehension, dread animals, of busy streets, of Crowd, in a Dark, of dogs, of examination, before examination, of failure, of health of loved persons, about narrow Places, in Vaults, Churches and cellars for a long time, Fear of Spiders.
27. Forgetful.
28. Gestures; tapping on's Skull with his fingers.
29. Grief, can not cry.
30. Grimaces.
31. Horrible things; affect her profoundly.

32. Idiocy; Mongols.
33. Indifference; apathy to loved ones.
34. Industrious; because he can not stand that he is reproached. That affects him to deeply.
35. Irritability; morning; after rising; because of forgetfulness.
36. Memory; Weakness Of, For everybody things.
37. Mistakes; While reading.
38. Music; aggravates; ameliorates or aversion to
39. Obstinate;
40. Offended easily;
41. Precocity:
42. Read, Passion to read, lectophile.
43. Remorse;
44. Reproaches; ailments from, others.
45. Sadness, in Children
46. Restlessness, Children in.
47. Schizophrenia.
48. Sensitive; oversensitive to Music, to Noise, to Reprimands.
49. Shrieking, Screaming, Night.
50. Starting, Sleep, From.
51. Suicidal; disposition; cancer history in the Family, with.
52. Suspicious, Mistrustful.
53. Sympathy, Comment for Animals only.
54. Talks, adult, like a- lawyer, like a, in a Child.
55. Thunderstorm, loves.
56. Tidy.
57. Timidity; School Children.

58. Touch everything, impelled to (Children).
59. Travel, desire to.
60. Unfortunate, Feels.
61. Unhappiness, prolonged, due to other People influence.
62. Weeping, admonitions, from music, when telling of her sickness.
63. Inquisitive.
64. Anxiety fits.

HEAD

1. Constriction, Tension.
2. Heaviness, Forehead, open air ameliorates.
3. Injuries of the head, after.
4. Pain; afternoon; 1 to 6 p.m; Pulsating; Deep inside the head; during or before thunderstorm. Pain forehead; Pulsating, extending to eyes, above right eye, behind. One sided- right side, pressing right temple. Pulsating, deep-seated, occiput.

EYE

1. Blueness, Conjunctiva, Sclerae.
2. Discolouration, blue (Porcelain) Sclerae.
3. Pain; Sore, lids, Margins of. Stinging Upper Lids.
4. Styes.
5. Twitching, lower lids, left; Eyebrows.
6. Winking.
7. Weak.

EAR

1. Eruptions, boils, inside, alternating one ear to the other.
2. Inflammation, Inside (Metal Wall, Right lobe).
3. Stopped. (Blocked Sensation).

NOSE

1. Coryza, frequent, tendency to.
2. Discharge, Excoriating.

FACE

1. Discolouration; bluish, lips; brown (Coffee Coloured); Café au lait Complexion and moles.
2. Eruptions, acne.
3. Heat, flushes, Climaxis, during.
4. Stiffness, lower jaw; paralytic.
5. Twitching.

MOUTH

1. Lump, Sensation.
2. Pain, Gums; Pressure. Sore palate.
3. Papillae, tongue, absent at tip.
4. Speech, Stammering.
5. Taste, putrid.
6. Ulcers.

TEETH

1. Biting, Nails, Fingers, gently the tips of Children's fingers.

2. Pain, aching.

THROAT

1. Inflammation, Tonsils, Chronic.
2. Lump, Plug, Etc., Sensation of.
3. Pain, evening aggravates.
4. Cold drink ameliorates.
5. Swallowing, empty, aggravates, when not warm drinks aggravates. Sore throat aggravated in morning and at night.
6. Scraping, Speak, before able to.
7. Induration of glands.

STOMACH

1. Anxiety.
2. Appetite, wanting.
3. Desires; Chocolate; Meat, fat, fat meat, seasoned food, alcoholic drinks, cold drinks.
4. Aversions; Fruit.
5. Desires; Soup
6. Constriction.
7. Eructations.
8. Indigestion.
9. Nausea, while riding in a carriage.
10. Pain, Coughing.
11. Ulcers (Ulcer Pepticum); with a strong family history.
12. Vomiting; alternating with diarrhoea periodic (Cyclical).

ABDOMEN

1. Constriction.
2. Emptiness, Sinking feeling in the region of umbilicus.
3. Enlarged, liver.
4. Flatulence.
5. Pain, in afternoon, at 4 to 6 p.m. bending double ameliorates. Pain from Constipation. Ameliorated by pressure, warm drinks. Digging pain above the region of umbilicus which comes and goes slowly.
6. Ulcers (ulcer pepticum).

RECTUM

1. Constipation; ineffectual urging and straining.
2. Constriction; ameliorated by bending.
3. Diarrhoea; Children.
4. Haemorrhage; from anus.
5. Inactivity, of rectum.
6. Pain, amelioration from pressure and warm drinks.
7. Prolapsus; Children Worms, Complaints of.

STOOL

1. Dry. Hard.

URINE

1. Albuminous. Casts, granular.

MALE

1. Erection, wanting.
2. Masturbation; disposition to in Children.

FEMALE

1. Masturbation, disposition.
2. Menopause.
3. Tumors, Uterus.

LARYNX AND TRACHEA

1. Lump Like Sensation in Larynx.

RESPIRATION

1. Asthmatic; From Fright.
2. Difficult; after, running.

COUGH

1. Morning, dressing while.
2. Evening, 8 to 11 p.m.
3. Air, Cold.
4. From, bathing, eating, inspiration, laughing, shaving, singing, talking.
5. Stomach, Seems to Come From.
6. Tickling, in Throat pit, From night.
7. Uncovering; dressing aggravates.
8. Warm room, Entering, from open air. Going from, to Cold air, or Vice-versa aggravates.

9. Whooping, Cough (Prolonged); early in life.
10. Yawning.

CHEST

1. Cancer, Mammae.
2. Constriction, Sensation of, Heart, Sight, as if wants to.
3. Eruption, Sternum, Undressing aggravates.
4. Inflammation, Lungs, Chronic, infants, Mammae, Chronic.
5. Oppression, inspiration, desire for deep.
6. Pain, Sternum, behind, Stitching, heart, Standing.
7. Palpitation, Heart, Afternoon, 2 to 6 p.m. audible, lying down aggravates. Extending to ear. Tumultuous, violent Palpitation. Visible palpitation.

BACK

1. Eruptions, dorsal region, Shoulders, between. Undressing aggravates.
2. Formication.
3. Pain, Cervical region, right, on turning head. (to right). dorsal region, scapulae, left.
4. Inner angle of Sacral region.
5. Twitching.

EXTREMITIES

1. Coldness, air, draft of.
2. Hangnails:
3. Heaviness, upper limbs, sudden.

4. Numbness, Thigh, effort, Physical Marked ameliorates. Sleep, short ameliorates.
5. Pain, rheumatic, lower limb Sciatica, leg motion (quick) aggravates. (Slow) ameliorates. Rheumatic warmth ameliorates aching, shoulder motion ameliorates, warmth ameliorates. Thigh effort, physical, marked ameliorates. Sleep, short ameliorates.
6. Twitching.
7. Varices, lower limbs.
8. Weakness, thigh; effort, physical, marked, ameliorates. Sleep, short ameliorates.

SLEEP

1. Disturbed.
2. Dreams; exciting, Journeys (drifting); Looking for Someone (and failing to find them). Murder; Nightmares; rousing the patient; snakes; work.
3. Restless.
4. Short, refreshes.
5. Sleeplessness; evening, after going to bed. Midnight, after, 4 hr. Children, in nursing, in rocked, child must be rocked, thoughts, from activity of walking after.
6. Unrefreshing.

SKIN

1. Discoloration; brown (Coffee-Coloured).
2. Eruptions, Eczema, in Children.
3. Moles; Naevi.
4. Keloid.

GENERALITIES

1. Afternoon, (13-18 h); (17-18 h)
2. Evening, (18- 21 h) (18-19 h)
3. Night
4. Acidosis.
5. Air, open ameliorates, sea- shore aggravates. or ameliorates.
6. Anaemia, pernicious (in family history).
7. Cancerous affections; cachexia, emaciation with aims, to relief.
8. Change, Symptoms, Constant Chronic of.
9. Children, affections in biting nails.
10. Cold, aggravation or amelioration.
11. Air ameliorates.
12. Heat and Cold.
13. Tendency to take cold.
14. Collapse.
15. Constriction, Sensation of external.
16. Contradictory and alternating states.
17. Dwarfishness.
18. Good health before diseases, Paroxysm.
19. Haemorrhage, orifices of the body, from.
20. Heat, Flushes of, Climacteric.
21. Inflammation, Hepatitis, Sinusitis, Tonsillitis.
22. Irritability; lack of.
23. Lassitude.
24. Masturbation, onanism, from.

25. Mononucleosis infectiosa, acute. After- effects from; never well since.
26. Mucous Secretions, acrid, thick.
27. Old People.
28. Pain, burning (internally); Sharp, tearing; (Internally).
29. Periodicity, annually.
30. Pulsation; internally.
31. Reaction; lack of.
32. Shuddering; waking on.
33. Sides; alternating; crosswise.
34. Sleep; Short Sleep ameliorates.
35. Tumors; Keloid, Cheloid.
36. Twitching; Waking on.
37. Undressing; agg; after.
38. Vaccination, after
39. Varicose veins.
40. Vaults, Cellars, agg.
41. Warm; agg; amel; room agg.
42. Weariness.
43. Weather; storm, during, amel; after.
44. Whooping-Cough; ailments after

Bibliography

B. JAIN PUBLISHERS (P) LTD.

1. Allen, JH 2002, *The Chronic Miasms Psora & Sycosis,* B. Jain Publishers (P) Ltd., New Delhi, India
2. Allen, H.C, *The Materia Medica of The Nosodes Proving of the X-ray,* B. Jain Publishers (P) Ltd., New Delhi
3. Allen, TF *1997, Encyclopedia of pure Materia Medica,* 11th edn,, B. Jain Publishers (P) Ltd., New Delhi, India.
4. Banerjea, S.K. *Miasmatic Diagnosis,* B. Jain Publishers (P) Ltd., New Delhi
5. Banerjee, P N *Chronic Disease - Its Cause and Cure,* B. Jain Publishers (P) Ltd., New Delhi
6. Boenninghausen, 2003, *The Lesser Writings of C. M. F Boenninghausen,* Translated by Prof. L. H. Tafel, Reprint edn,, B. Jain Publishers (P) Ltd., New Delhi, India
7. Boericke/Dudgeon *Organon 5th and 6th ed. Hahnemann,* B. Jain Publishers (P) Ltd., New Delhi
8. Brewster O'Reilly *Organon of the Medical Art by Dr. Samuel Hahnemann (ed. by Brewster O'Reilly),* B. Jain Publishers (P) Ltd., New Delhi

9. Burnett, James Compton *The Best of Burnett,* B. Jain Publishers (P) Ltd., New Delhi

10. Choudhury, HM 2005, *Indications of Miasms,* 2nd edn, B. Jain Publishers (P) Ltd., New Delhi, India

11. Close, S 2004, *The Genius of Homoeopathy; Lectures and Essays on Homoeopathic Philosophy,* 1st edn, B. Jain Publishers (P) Ltd., New Delhi, India.

12. Dudgeon, RE 2002, *Lectures on Theory and Practice of Homoeopathy,* reprint edn, B.Jain Publishers, New Delhi.

13. Hahnemann Samuel *Chronic Diseases Theoretical Part,* B. Jain Publishers (P) Ltd., New Delhi

14. Hahnemann Samuel *Lesser Writings of Samuel Hahnemann,* B. Jain Publishers (P) Ltd., New Delhi

15. Hering, C 1997, *Guiding Symptoms of our Materia Medica,* 1st edn,, B. Jain Publishers (P) Ltd., New Delhi, India.

16. Julian,O.A. *Materia Medica of Nosodes with Repertory,* B. Jain Publishers (P) Ltd., New Delhi

17. Kent, JT 2004, *Lectures on Homeopathic Philosophy,* 1st edn,, B. Jain Publishers (P) Ltd., New Delhi, India

18. Kent, J.T. *Lesser Writings,* B. Jain Publishers (P) Ltd., New Delhi

19. Koehler, G. (1986) *The Handbook of Homoeopathy,* B. Jain Publishers (P) Ltd., New Delhi

20. Master, Farokh *Tubercular Miasm,* B. Jain Publishers (P) Ltd., New Delhi

21. Mathur, K.N. *Principles of Prescribing,* B. Jain Publishers (P) Ltd., New Delhi

22. Nigam, Harsh Dr. 2008 *Principles and Practice of Homoeopathic Case Management,* B. Jain Publishers (P) Ltd., New Delhi

23. Ortega, P.S. 1980 *Notes on Miasms,* Ist English Edition National Homoeopathic Pharmacy Hanuman Road,New Delhi India

24. Roberts, HA 2005, *The principal and Art of Cure by Homoeopathy,* 3rd edn,, B. Jain Publishers New Delhi

25. Sankaran, Rajan *Homoeopathy, The Science of Healing,* B. Jain Publishers (P) Ltd., New Delhi

26. Tyler, M.L *Hahnemann's Conception of Chronic Diseases,* B. Jain Publishers (P) Ltd., New Delhi

OTHER PUBLICATIONS

27. Agrawal, Y.R., *Comparative Study of Chronic Miasms,* Vijay Publications, Delhi

28. Fortier-Bernoville & Nebel, *Tuberculinsm,* London Publishing House

29. Foubister *Tutorials on Homeopathy,* Beaconsfield Publishers Ltd., Beaconsfield

30. Geukens, A.; Mortelmans,G *Carcinosin.* Vzw Centrum Voor Homoeopathie, Belgium, Hechtel eksch Belgium. 1989

31. Ian Watson *A Guide to the Methodologies,* Cutting Edge Publications, Devon

32. Klaus D. Elgert *Immunology: Understanding the Immune System* Medical 2009

33. Paschero T.P., *Homeopathy,* Elsevier.

34. Sankran P., *Some Notes On Nosodes* Homoeopathic Medical Publications, Bombay 1978

35. Speight Phyllis; *A Comparison Of Chronic Miasms*, Rustington/ Sussex 1961

36. Vinay Kumar, Stanley L Robbins, *Robbins Basic Pathology*, Saunders/Elsevier, 2007

JOURNALS

37. Elizabeth Wright, *The Problem of Suppression*, The Homoeopathic Recorder Vol. XLIV no.10 1929, pg 693Foubister D.M.

38. Foubister, D.M., *The Carcinosin Drug Picture,* The British Homoeopathic Journal, Vol. XLVII No.3, 1958, Pg 202

39. Foubister, D.M., *Indications For Certain Nosodes,* The British Homoeopathic Journal, Vol. XXXIX No.3, 1939, Pg 269

40. Gibson, *Psorinum A Study*, The British Homoeopathic Journal, Vol. XIXVIVIII No.3, 1968, Pg 192

41. Goldberg, *The Nosodes in Homoeotherapeutics,* The Journal Of The American Institute of Homeopathy No.3

42. H, Montfort-Cabello, *Chronic Disease: What Are They?*; Homeopathy Vol.93 Issue 2, April 2004.

43. Hatfield, *Thoughts On Miasma in Practice*, The British Homoeopathic Journal, Vol. XXVIII No.3, 1938, Pg 251

44. Leddermann, E.K., *Homoeopathy and The Existential Phenomenological Approach,* The British Homoeopathic Journal, Vol. XIXVI No.3, 1966, Pg 251

45. Mecislao solvey, *A Modern Look at Carcinosins*, The Journal Of The American Institute of Homeopathy No.3, Vol. 68 1975 Pg 159

46. Paschero, T.P.: *Psora, Idiosyncrasy Fundamental of Pathology;* Hahnemannian Gleanings, 1960

47. Paschero, T.P.: *Tuberculinum;* Hahnemannian Gleanings, 1960
48. Patterson, Elisabeth: *A survey of Nosodes*, The British Homoeopathic Journal, Vol. XLIX No.3, 1960, Pg 224
49. Speight Phyllis, *Homoeopathy and The Miasm*, The Homoeopathic World Vol. 100 No.1 1962 pg
50. Nigam, Harsh; *Immunity and Homoeopathy;* Sharnam Homeopathic Research Society 1998.